The Emergency Pantry Handbook

How to Prepare Your Family for Just about Everything

Kate Rowinski

Photography by Jim Rowinski

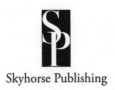

Skyhorse Publishing

Skyhorse Publishing books may be purchased in bulk at special discounts for sales promotion, corporate gifts, fund-raising, or educational purposes. Special editions can also be created to specifications. For details, contact the Special Sales Department, Skyhorse Publishing, 307 West 36th Street, 11th Floor, New York, NY 10018 or info@skyhorsepublishing.com.

Skyhorse® and Skyhorse Publishing® are registered trademarks of Skyhorse Publishing, Inc.®, a Delaware corporation.

www.skyhorsepublishing.com

10 9 8 7 6 5 4 3

Library of Congress Cataloging-in-Publication Data is available on file.

ISBN: 978-1-62087-590-2

Printed in the United States of America.

Contents

Introduction

Why Do You Need a Food Pantry?

In this uncertain day and age, it seems that potential disasters lurk around every corner—wild weather, the threat of terrorism, economic concerns—it is easy to feel that you and your family could fall victim at any moment. Ask yourself these questions: What if we lose power or the water is shut off? What if I lose my income? Could I feed my family for a day, a week, even a month? What if access to grocery stores was unavailable? Do I have a way to store and cook food in my home?

With fast food and easy access to almost anything, it may be hard to imagine a world of scarcity. But the reality is that scarcity can happen in an instant. A large tree falling on a road may keep you from the store for a day. A power outage may keep the stores closed for a week. Job loss may prevent you from shopping for three months or more.

You don't have to be a doomsday believer or a radical survivalist to consider creating your own emergency food pantry. In fact, the idea of not having a back-up supply of food should be as nonsensical to you as not having a tank of gas or extra batteries.

Rather than allowing the specter of disaster to loom in the back of your mind, there are simple steps you can take to make sure that your family's basic needs can be taken care of in the event of an emergency. Establishing a food plan gives you the following benefits:

A Powerful Insurance Policy

Food storage is the most powerful of all bank accounts, allowing you to get through any lean times without desperation or handouts. Knowing that you have what you need no matter what happens can give you peace of mind that no homeowner's policy could ever provide.

A Sense of Self-Sufficiency

Knowing that you can take care of yourself and your family has a powerful effect on your psychological state. Taken even further, understanding how to grow and preserve your own food will give your family greater appreciation for where their food comes from and a sense of gratitude for what they have.

Helping Others

Did you know the average family has less than a week's worth of food in their kitchen right now? And worse yet, if there was no power, many people wouldn't even know how to cook it! Your food pantry and cooking plan will not only help keep your family safe, but may allow you to help others as well.

Not long ago, a hurricane knocked out power to our area, taking down trees that prevented us from getting out for a few days. We were astonished to learn that most of our neighbors were not prepared to do something as simple as heating a can of beans. They could have gotten by on cereal or cheese and crackers for a couple of days, but many relied entirely on electric ranges and some had outdoor grills that were out of propane. Worst of all, many had no emergency water stored. It's not that they were completely without resources; they just didn't have a plan.

But what could have been a very uncomfortable situation turned into a party. People contributed food out of their now-useless freezers, and our emergency cooking plan fed the whole neighborhood for three days. We distributed gallons of drinking water and a neighbor with a swimming pool supplied water for toilets.

So how do you plan for unexpected events?

o———————o

Establish Your Goals

Creating a food pantry may seem like a daunting task. Dedicated space is needed, time is required, both to gather supplies and to maintain them, and you have to be able to afford the necessary supplies to get started. So first take the time to determine what you want to accomplish.

Establish how much money and space can be allocated to your food storage project. It is important to take stock before rushing out and buying supplies willy-nilly. It is not necessary to create a millennial plan in order to begin, but it isn't enough to just run out and buy extra food. If you aren't ready for a big commitment, just start out with a carefully planned three-day supply of food and water. Even this small step will put you ahead of most of your neighbors. You will find that a lot of the components that go into being self-sufficient for three days are the same things that you need for longer term planning. So go slowly and get it right in the beginning. You will end up with a better plan all around.

As you grow comfortable with the planning process, it will be time to expand your pantry to include long-term storage. Again, think about your goal. Consider the degree of self-sufficiency you are seeking. Even if you think you want a one-year supply of food, start by working on your three-month plan first. Remember, a large supply of food requires care and rotation; it's not enough to just go out and buy a lot of food.

Once you have committed to the size and scope of your pantry, you are ready to get into the details. Chapters 3 and 4 will take you through the process of planning and execution.

One Step at a Time

Emergency food planning is not an all-or-nothing proposition. As soon as you start to think ahead, you will quickly find that every step you take, no matter how small, gives you more control over your situation than you had before.

Begin by stocking a three-day supply of food for your family. Make sure you include nutritious items that don't require refrigeration or cooking.

Store water! Have at least three gallons on hand for each member of the family.

Slowly build your supply of staples and family favorites so that you could comfortably get by for two weeks.

o———————o

Assess Your Resources

How much space is available for food storage? There is no point in making a one-year plan if your storage is going to be limited to a spare closet. Look around your home and think creatively, keeping in mind that the location you choose should be dry with a reasonably consistent temperature. Damp basements, freezing garages, or hot attics are not good choices.

What are your cooking arrangements if energy sources are limited? Take stock of your home. Is there a fireplace or wood stove that could be pressed into service? If not, do you have outdoor space for propane or charcoal cooking? What kinds of food would you need if no cooking was possible?

Next, think about how you will provide food for your family. Will your pantry satisfy all your needs, or will your plan include bartering or growing your own food and learning to preserve it? Again, assess your resources. Do you have a sunny location for growing vegetables? You don't need a large yard to grow your own food, and even a patio can provide fresh greens or herbs. There are great small-space options that produce high yields.

o———————o

Take Action!

Your goals are set, your storage location is chosen, and you have some ideas on alternative cooking sources. Now is the time to act!

You don't have to wait until you have a lot of extra money to get started creating your storage pantry. If you set aside as little as $10 a week from your grocery bill to devote to your pantry, you will see great dividends in short order. I am a big fan of the weekly specials at my local store, where I can load up on beans and canned tomatoes, as well as boxed macaroni and cheese, and other family favorites.

Of course, if you are a coupon clipper, you can find great deals. Just make sure to stick to your list! You don't want to suddenly find yourself with a five-year supply of something that was on sale but may be impractical for long-term storage!

1

Preparing Your Family for an Emergency

Before launching into your full-blown food storage plan, make sure that you have taken all the necessary steps to be ready should an emergency strike. This means knowing where to meet, how you'll communicate, what resources you have for heating and transportation, and how to handle the basic functions of your home. Take the time to create your plans and walk the entire family through them. It's not enough for you to know what to do; other members of the household need to know, too!

Make a Family Plan

Many of us who were around on 9/11 realized (after the fact) just how vulnerable we were when it came to reaching out to family and friends in the middle of an emergency. Phone lines may be jammed, networks may be down, and confusion can quickly turn to panic.

With work, school, and a myriad of other activities, chances are that your family may not be together if a disaster strikes. That's why it is so important to plan in advance. Get your family together and discuss your emergency plan:

How will you know if there is an emergency? State and local agencies may have alerts available that you can register for simply by providing your

1

email address. Likewise, the National Oceanic and Atmospheric Administration (NOAA) issues regular weather alerts.

What is your safe place? If your home is not an option due to storm or fire, agree to meet somewhere else that everyone in the family is familiar with.

How will you contact one another? Cell service may not be available, so what are your other options? Be sure every member of your family carries important phone numbers with them and has coins, or a prepaid phone card to call their emergency contacts.

In a local emergency, it is often easier to call out-of-state than it is to call across town. Identify a friend or relative who lives out-of-state and who everyone can notify that they are safe.

If you have a cell phone, program your emergency contact as "ICE" (In Case of Emergency) in your phone. If you are in an accident, emergency personnel will check for an ICE listing in your contacts folder in order to get a hold of someone you know. Make sure to tell your family and friends that you've listed them as emergency contacts. In addition, do the following:

- Teach children to call 911.
- Keep a collar, license, and I.D. on your dog at all times.
- Make sure everyone in the family knows how to use text messaging. Text messages can often get through when a phone call cannot.
- Include neighbors in your plan. Identify safe houses for your children that they can go to in case parents are unable to get home.
- Write down your plan and keep a copy of it in your safe or a fireproof box so you can access it in the event of a disaster. Adults should keep a copy in their wallets or handbags, and children can have a copy in a school pack or taped to the inside of a notebook.

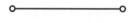

Organize

In this tech-friendly world, it is tempting to keep track of many of your most important accounts and policies online. But in the event of an emergency, life can quickly get frustrating without important contacts and policy numbers at the ready.

Buy a small home safe or fireproof box and create a comprehensive list of everything you might need to know in the event of an emergency. Your safe should include the following:

- Copies of each of your credit cards (front and back).
- All of your insurance policies, along with contact name and number of your agent.
- Copy of all driver's licenses, car titles, and passports.
- Photo identification of children and birth certificates.
- Animal registration, vaccination records, and photo identification of your pet.
- List of doctors' names, addresses, and telephone numbers.
- List of all family medical prescriptions, with strength of dosage.
- A list of any important valuables. Keep a video record of every room in your house, boats, and other vehicles so that you can refer to them for insurance purposes.
- Ready cash in small denominations, including coins.

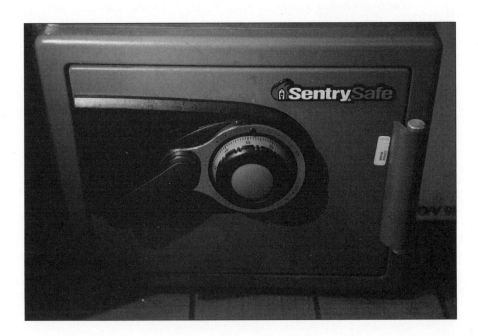

How much cash do I need?

Ask any expert about cash reserves and their advice will be about the same. Keep three to six months' worth of expenses readily available. Put this money in a regular savings account, not locked up in a CD or other non-liquid account where withdrawing early will cost you a penalty. Calculate your total bills and other essential expenses such as food and gas and use that as your baseline. You can round up or down, based on your own comfort level. But remember, liquid assets don't earn much interest, so don't go overboard and keep all your assets liquid.

As to actual cash, we use the three-day rule. We try to keep enough cash in our home safe to get by for three days in case we have to leave the house suddenly due to a fire or other natural disaster. The amount of money to keep handy is to cover food, gas, hotel rooms, or other emergency needs such as extra clothes or toiletries. For us, that figure is about $1,000. If that amount sounds like too much, calculate your own figure.

Keep an assortment of bills in your home stash. If the power is out and stores are unable to run their registers, a nice supply of one and five dollar bills will be very handy. Keep your money in a home safe or fireproof box along with your other important papers.

Do a Home Inventory

Is your house ready for any emergency? Walk through your house and yard and ask yourself the following questions:

- Are smoke detectors installed on every level of the house and are batteries current?
- Do you have a working wired landline phone?
- Are battery-operated devices all in working order?

- Are mirrors and heavy pictures well-secured?
- Are hallways and other exits clear and uncluttered?
- Are bookshelves secured to the wall, with heavy items on the lowest shelves?
- Is there a fire extinguisher on each level and do you know how to use it?
- Are flammable or highly reactive chemicals such as bleach, ammonia, and paint thinners stored safely and out of the reach of children?
- Do you know how to turn off water and gas mains and shut down electricity?
- Are sump pumps working? Are generators or other emergency devices in good working order?
- Do all doors and windows have working locks?
- Is your house number visible from the street?
- Are there any trees, limbs, utility poles, or other objects that could cause safety issues?
- Are drainage outlets, eaves troughs, and gutters clear?
- Is there charcoal or extra propane for the outdoor grills?

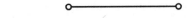

Create a Home Emergency Kit

Natural disasters can cause a lot of chaos, and even with the best possible plans in place, it may take emergency personnel a few days to reach everyone and make supplies available.

So what does your family need to get by? Your emergency kit should be designed to last for a minimum of three days and include the following:

- Water. You will need about one gallon of water per person per day for drinking and sanitation.
- Food. You will want at least a three-day supply of non-perishable food that requires minimal or no cooking. If you have babies, make sure formula and diapers are included.
- Manual can opener for opening canned items.
- One flashlight with batteries for every family member.
- One larger fluorescent lantern for illuminating a whole room.

- An LED headlamp, useful for hands-free damage assessment and repairs.
- Battery-operated radio and clock.
- Extra batteries.
- A cooler and ice for items you will need easy access to, like baby formula or refrigerated medicine.
- List of important phone numbers.
- First aid kit, along with important prescription medications. When I get new prescription glasses, I add my old ones to the kit.
- An extra set of car keys.
- Emergency shelter including plastic sheeting or tarps, and duct tape to repair walls or create shelter-in-place.
- Moist towelettes and garbage bags for personal sanitation.
- A basic tool kit, including hammer, screwdriver, wrench, and utility knife.
- Local maps.
- Cell phone with home and car charger or solar charger.
- Sleeping bag or warm blanket for each person.
- Complete change of clothing including a long sleeve shirt, long pants, and sturdy shoes.
- Household chlorine bleach and medicine dropper. When diluted, nine parts water to one part bleach, can be used as a disinfectant.

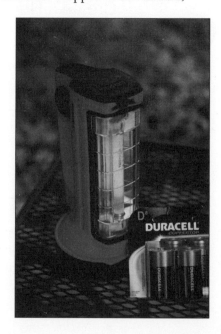

- Spare tank of propane for outdoor cooking.
- Fire extinguisher.
- Paper and pencil and a supply of books, games, playing cards, or puzzles.

Choose a cool, dry location to store your emergency supplies. Label food items with the date you are placing them in storage. Keep food in tightly closed plastic containers to keep out rodents, insects, and excess moisture. Place sleeping bags and spare clothing in plastic garbage bags. Tools and other gear can be stored together in another large plastic container. We use five-gallon plastic buckets to store all our supplies.

Maintain your supplies by refreshing them every six months or so. Check dates and discard old items.

Label water containers and replace drinking water with fresh containers. Think about any new or different needs and add to your kit accordingly.

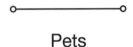

Pets

Some of the most heartbreaking sights of Hurricane Katrina were the faces of lost and stranded animals. When disaster strikes, it may feel like all you can do is get yourself ready, but the animals in your life are counting on you for protection, so take a little time to get them ready, too.

- Place a rescue alert sticker on the window of your home so emergency workers know that animals may be inside the house.
- Make sure your pet's collar has current address tags and updated immunization tags. Even better, have your vet insert a microchip. Most animal shelters can scan for microchips so pets can be identified even if they lose their collars.
- Have a bug-out pack ready for them, containing all the items they will need to survive away from home. This will include a leash and an extra collar, three to seven days worth of food and water, feeding bowl, blanket, and crate.
- Photocopy veterinary and immunization records; if you have to shelter the dog in a kennel, you will need to provide evidence of health. Include photographs of the pet in case it gets lost.
- Arrange for a safe shelter for your pet in the event that you have to leave them behind. Locate recommended kennels in other cities, arrange with a friend or family member who can take them, and know what hotels will accept pets.
- Keep a leash near the door at all times in case you need to make a hasty exit. If bad weather threatens, make sure to keep pets in the house. Bad weather can upset pets, and they may hide or even run off if they become disoriented.

○────────○

Create a Car Emergency Kit

Keep items in the car in case of an emergency. Never run your car on fumes. There should always be at least half a tank of gas in your car at all times. If you have an appropriate way to store it, consider keeping two weeks' worth of fuel available for your car. This kit should include:

- Three-day supply of food items containing protein, such as nuts and energy bars
- Three-day supply of water
- Emergency blankets
- Warm clothes, gloves, hat, sturdy boots, jacket, and an extra change of clothes
- Flashlights and extra batteries
- Jumper cables
- Cell phone charger
- An LED headlamp
- First aid kit and necessary medication
- AM/FM radio
- Cat litter or sand for better tire traction
- Shovel and ice scraper
- Basic car tools, including jack, lug wrench, tow chain, and spare parts
- Flares
- Cash

○────────○

Pre-Built Emergency Kits

There are a number of good pre-built kits on the market today, designed specifically for emergency use. They generally hold water, purification tablets, and protein bars, along with flashlights, space blanket, basic tools, and first aid supplies.

○────────○

The Three-Day Food Plan

Whether you are interested in long-term emergency food storage or not, everyone should have an emergency plan that includes enough easy-to-cook food to last for three days. The good news is that three days' worth of food can fit comfortably into a little-used cupboard, a closet, in bins under the bed, even in an alcove under the stairs. The location you choose should be cool and dry, without direct sunlight. Take note of appliances or pipes that can overheat small spaces.

Your plan should include the following for *each person* in your household. Caloric requirements vary, based on size and activity levels, but figure everyone needs between 1,600 and 2,800 calories per day.

- One gallon of potable water per person per day.
- Grains: A minimum of eighteen servings of grains, breads, rice, or pasta; at least six servings per day per person.
- Fruit: A minimum of six servings of any type of fruit, avocados, or tomatoes; at least two servings per day per person.
- Vegetables: A minimum of nine servings of any type of vegetable; at least three servings per day per person.
- Protein: A minimum of six servings of any type of meat, legumes, eggs, peanut butter, or nuts; at least two servings per day per person.
- Dairy: A minimum of six servings of milk, yogurt, or cheese; at least two servings per day per person.

Daily Servings			
	Low	**Moderate**	**High**
	Sedentary Women Older Adults	Most Children Teen Girls Active Women Pregnant and Nursing Women Sedentary Men	Teen Boys Active Men
Calories	1,600	2,200	2,800
Water	1 gallon	1 gallon	1 gallon
Grains	6	9	11
Vegetables	3	4	5
Fruit	2	3	4
Dairy	2–3	2–4	2–5
Meat	2	2	2

A three-day emergency menu might look something like this:

Day 1	Day 2	Day 3
Breakfast	**Breakfast**	**Breakfast**
Granola with milk and canned peaches	Oatmeal with brown sugar, nuts, raisins, and milk	Pancakes with syrup Stewed apples
Lunch	**Lunch**	**Lunch**
Split pea soup Cornbread	Tuna salad with brown bread	Tomato soup Cheese and rye crackers
Dinner	**Dinner**	**Dinner**
Angel hair pasta with spaghetti sauce, white beans, and spinach	Rice Refried black beans Corn	Brown rice and lentils Canned peas

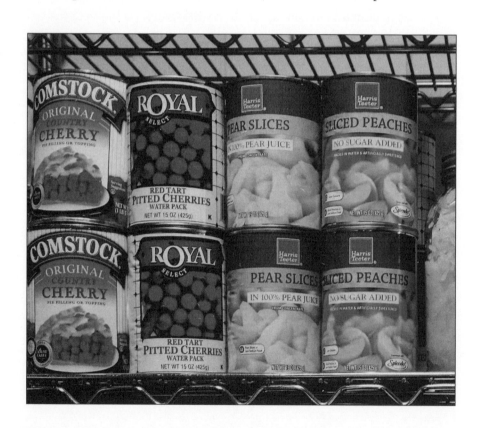

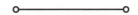

When the Power Goes Out

Refrigerated Food

Most refrigerated foods that are held above 40°F for more than two hours should be considered suspect. If a major power outage lasts more than about four hours, it is likely that most of your refrigerated food will have to be discarded. There are a few exceptions, like hard cheeses, some prepared foods, and most fresh produce. Inspect each item individually for signs of mold or staleness, and discard anything that doesn't look or smell good.

See the chart below for USDA recommendations.

REFRIGERATED FOODS: KEEP OR DISCARD?	
KEEP	**DISCARD**
MEATS AND PROTEINS	**MEATS AND PROTEINS**
	Raw or leftover cooked meat, poultry, fish, or seafood
	Soy meat substitutes, tofu
	Thawing meat or poultry
	Meat, tuna, shrimp, chicken, or egg salads
	Gravy, stuffing, broth
	Lunchmeats, hot dogs, bacon, sausage, dried beef
	Canned hams labeled "Keep Refrigerated"
	Canned meats and fish, opened
	Casseroles, soups, stews
DAIRY	**DAIRY**
Hard Cheeses: cheddar, Swiss, provolone	Soft Cheeses
Processed cheeses	Shredded Cheeses

Continued on next page

Parmesan, Romano, whole or grated	Low-fat cheeses
Butter, margarine	Milk and milk products
	Baby formula, opened
	Fresh eggs, hard-cooked in shell, egg dishes, egg products
	Custards and puddings, quiche
FRUITS	**FRUITS**
Fresh fruit juices, opened	Fresh fruits, cut
Fresh canned fruits, opened	
Fresh fruits, coconut, raisins, dried fruits, candied fruits, dates	
SAUCES AND CONDIMENTS	**SAUCES AND CONDIMENTS**
Jelly, relish, taco sauce, mustard, catsup, olives, pickles	Opened mayonnaise, tartar sauce, horseradish
Worcestershire, soy, barbecue, hoisin sauces	Opened cream-based dressings
Opened vinegar-based dressings	Spaghetti sauce, opened jar
	Fish sauces, oyster sauce
PACKAGED PRODUCTS	**PACKAGED PRODUCTS**
Peanut butter	Refrigerator biscuits, rolls, cookie dough
Bread, rolls, cakes, muffins, quick breads, tortillas	Cooked pasta, rice, potatoes
Breakfast foods (waffles, pancakes, bagels)	Pasta salads with mayonnaise or vinaigrette
Pies, fruit	Fresh pasta
	Cheesecake
	Pastries, cream filled
	Pies (custard, cheese filled, or chiffon; quiche)
VEGETABLES	**VEGETABLES**
Fresh mushrooms, herbs, spices	Greens, pre-cut, pre-washed, packaged

Vegetables, raw	Vegetables, cooked
	Vegetable juice, opened
	Baked potatoes
	Tofu
	Commercial garlic in oil
LEFTOVERS	**LEFTOVERS**
	Potato salad
	Casseroles, soups, stews
	Pizza, any topping
	Pasta salads with mayonnaise or vinaigrette

Frozen Food

Freezing is an easy and convenient way to preserve meat and homegrown produce. It is also very good for retaining the nutritional value of your food. The problem is that this storehouse of surplus food is dependent on the power staying on.

Food in the freezer will generally keep two to three days after the power goes out. There are a handful of things you can do to keep the cold in as long as possible.

- Choose a chest freezer over an upright one. Chest freezers retain their temperature longer.
- Avoid opening the freezer door unless absolutely necessary.
- Sort meats on one side of the freezer and other foods on the other side. That way, juices from meat products won't contaminate other foods. If you are expecting an outage, stack foods on top of one another to help them stay frozen longer.
- Don't run a half-empty freezer. It is inefficient and the food in there will melt even faster. If you have a lot of spare space in your freezer, fill milk or soda containers with water and place them in the freezer along with your other items. (Make sure to leave space in the bottles—water expands when frozen.) The extra ice will keep frozen foods cold longer. The other advantage is that this stored water provides another source of emergency drinking water.
- Thawed food should be used as soon as possible.

○────────────○

When You Can't Cook

Consider what your family would eat if no cooking sources were available. I keep canned brown bread, as well as a supply of high energy snacks such as nuts, peanut butter, crackers, protein bars, and trail mix handy. It also helps to have a few treats on hand, such as candy, pudding cups, or cocoa mix.

Another way to plan for this type of short-term emergency is by purchasing pre-cooked and packaged meals that have been freeze-dried or dehydrated. You can choose military-grade MREs (Meals Ready to Eat) that can be kept in storage for up to five years, or you can opt for an assortment of basic food stuffs that will last as long as twenty-five years.

2

Storing and Handling Water

Anyone who has lived through a power outage knows that water is not only critical for survival but is an essential element of the creature comforts we take for granted.

In spite of the discomfort hunger can cause, the reality is that most of us could get by days, and even weeks, without food. But we can't last a week without water. In fact, the average person in a reasonably comfortable environment and expending very little energy could probably only survive three to five days without water. Of course, flushing the toilet, cooking meals, and keeping clean also require a steady source of water.

How Much Water Do You Need?

A power outage or a freak storm can quickly throw your normal routine into a tailspin. Suddenly your pump won't work, and tap water will be just outside your grasp. Or worse, your public water supply becomes unavailable or non-potable. Floods and storms can damage or contaminate wells and municipal water systems, potentially making access to previously available resources out of the question for longer periods of time.

For these reasons, you should always have at least a three-day supply of potable drinking water for every person and animal in the household.

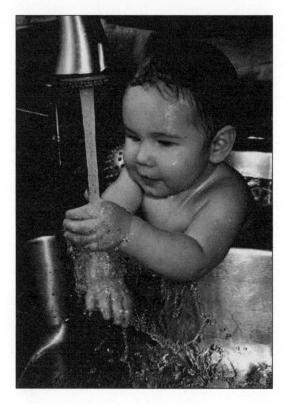

Children and small pets may be able to get by with a little less. That means that for a family of four, you should always have at least twelve gallons of bottled drinking water available. For cleaning and hygiene, another gallon per person would also be desirable.

Water is very heavy, which makes keeping a three-month supply rather daunting. That's ninety gallons per person, *just for drinking.* Plan another gallon per day for sanitation and personal needs.

Storing Water

Tap water is safe to store, so filling your own food-grade containers is a good way to get started. For large quantities of water, consider water storage barrels that can contain up to fifty-five gallons—enough for about a month for two people. Fifty-five-gallon food-quality drums are relatively easy to fill and store, but when full, they weigh over four hundred pounds. We prefer to store smaller containers, including five-gallon drums. Packaged water is available in every size imaginable, from personal bottle size to sealed five-gallon containers, and many of these can be re-used for water storage.

Keep water in a cool, dark place. Though freezing will not hurt it, it could cause overfilled containers to leak. Water does not have a definite shelf life, but it doesn't hurt to check large containers for cloudiness before use. Sealed containers should stay fresh indefinitely.

If your freezer is not full, consider keeping containers of water in there, too. Frozen water containers will help keep the freezer cold for longer, and provide an extra source of water as they melt. Just make sure to leave headroom to allow for containers to expand.

○————————○

Purifying Non-Potable Water

Water that has not been treated can contain organisms that may cause serious gastric distress. Water from lakes or streams, or rainwater in your

outdoor rain barrels, should always be treated before use. This applies to drinking water, as well as any water that you use to clean food, wash dishes, or brush your teeth.

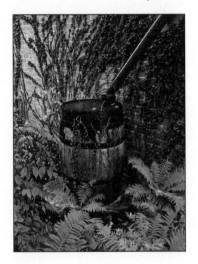

If water is cloudy or contains particulates, strain it before disinfecting it. Home water filters are not designed for disinfecting water but they may help to make your disinfected water more palatable, so it's a good idea to run it through your filter after boiling or bleaching it.

○————————○

Boiling

Bring water to a full rolling boil and let it boil for three to five minutes. Cool and store.

You may wish to keep sterilized water on hand for special purposes. Sterile water is useful for mixing infant formula or for cleaning wounds. To store sterilized water, bring a pot of water to a full boil. Clean and sterilize quart jars. Let the boiled water cool down enough to handle safely, and then fill the jars, leaving about an inch of headspace. Tighten lids and rings into place and process for about twenty-five minutes.

○────────────○

Disinfecting with Bleach

You can make water safe to drink by adding bleach. Bleach by itself is pretty toxic, so it is important to follow the instructions for purifying water exactly. Use only pure liquid bleach, not one that contains soap or any other ingredients. The label should say sodium hypochlorite. Most household bleaches come in a concentration of about 5–6 percent. To purify one gallon of water, add one-eighth teaspoon of bleach. For five gallons, place a half teaspoon (yes, that's all) into five gallons of water to purify it for drinking. If the water is cloudy, use twice that amount. Shake container to thoroughly incorporate bleach into the water. Let your treated water sit for at least forty-five minutes before using it to kill any bacteria that may be present.

The surprising thing about bleach is not how useful it is, but how little is actually needed to do the job. Here are some other great uses for bleach:

- Bleach is indispensable for removing mold and mildew. One cup of bleach in two gallons of water will remove stains from hard surfaces. Scrub, rinse, and repeat if necessary.
- Bleach makes a great disinfectant. Just mix one tablespoon of bleach with a gallon of water to clean almost anything.
- Sanitize dishes, glassware, and other items by soaking in one gallon of dishwater with a couple of tablespoons of bleach added. Ten minutes should do the trick. Rinse and air dry items in the sun.

○────────────○

Water for Hygiene

In addition to drinking water, you will want an available source of water for cleaning, maintaining your toilet, and basic hygiene. When storms threaten, simply filling the bathtub may give you the extra water you need for these basic tasks. Likewise, outdoor rain barrels are great for collecting this type of emergency water. Swimming pool or hot tub water may be handy for non-drinking purposes, like cleaning or flushing toilets. Because of the chemicals used in this type of water, avoid it as a source of drinking water.

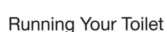

Running Your Toilet

There are two ways to use your toilet during a power outage. The first is to fill the toilet tank with water and flush as usual. The second way is simpler: just pour water directly into the bowl after use to flush down waste. Make sure to keep some water in the bowl at all times so fumes from the sewer or septic tank don't seep into the house. Only flush when absolutely necessary!

If you don't have enough water for running your toilet, there are camping toilets and even disposable bucket toilets designed for camping.

Laundry

Faced with days without power, you may wonder what happens when you run out of clean clothes. Hot water, a washtub, and scrubber will solve this problem, along with a heavy-duty clothesline. But a little forethought can keep the laundry from piling up too quickly.

For clothes that are not actually dirty, rather than tossing them in the laundry basket as you normally would, spray a little fabric freshener on them and hang them out in a well-ventilated place at the end of the day. Consider adding a t-shirt under your other clothes; this under layer can be washed more easily than a heavy sweatshirt. Keep certain clothes for messy tasks like cooking and change into those before you get started. If you do get a stain, stop and treat it immediately rather than changing clothes completely. A pen-style laundry stain remover can rescue a shirt for another day of use.

○────────────○

Personal Hygiene

Days without a shower can seem like torture for those of us accustomed to this everyday luxury. As long as you have enough water available, you can fashion a bath of sorts with hot water and soap. We keep wet wipes in our storage specifically for power outages. Not only does it save a lot of water, we find that using them for everything from washing faces and hands to substituting them for toilet paper keeps everyone feeling (relatively) fresh. Likewise, a squirt of liquid hand sanitizer allows you to avoid reaching for the water bottle unless you have something on your hands that really requires rinsing. A spray bottle of water can also go a long way after a hot or sweaty day.

Of course, nothing beats a good shower! We discovered the solar shower years ago when we started camping. This simple five-gallon PVC bag hangs in the sun where it can warm up water, and it comes with a small shower head.

○────────────○

Conserving Water

The first step in having enough water is knowing how to use it. We found this out the hard way one year when a particularly bad drought threatened our water supplies for several months. We learned in a hurry when and how to make the most of our water supply, how to find alternatives to running water, and how to collect and store it. We quickly replaced our high flow toilets with more efficient models and learned to stay clean with a minimum number of showers. Paper plates and plastic utensils became a lifesaver.

Before you have a water crisis, do an audit of your home to make sure you are doing all you can to conserve.

- Check faucets, pipes, and toilets for leaks.
- Install water-saving showerheads and toilets.

- Run the washing machine and dishwasher only when you have a full load.
- Learn to take shorter showers and shut off water while you brush your teeth or shave.
- Keep a bottle of cold water in the refrigerator instead of running tap water until it is cold.
- Outside, mulch plants to keep the soil around them moist. Use rain barrels or a rainwater tank to catch run-off.

3

Planning Your Long-Term Storage Pantry

Think of your long-term food storage plan as your "food bank account." You want that bank account to be a sound investment, one that you have ready access to, and one that will provide you with exactly what you need when you need it. Remember: No matter what a great deal it is, how long its shelf life, or how practical it might sound, there is absolutely no point in storing food you don't want to eat.

So what should go into your food pantry?

Eat What You Store and Store What You Eat

Build your own individualized food pantry using the common-sense "eat what you store, store what you eat" approach. This means that you only buy food you actually want to eat, food that your family is accustomed to, and food that you actually use every day, rather than accumulating it and locking it up tight for some future imagined time.

Because you are always rotating through your pantry, you don't have to wait for a full-scale emergency to use your food. You always have your own piggy bank to draw from, even when it's just a week where your budget is a little pinched.

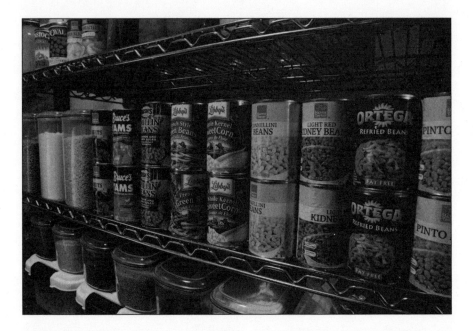

To start creating your own customized food pantry, consider the kinds of meals your family currently eats. Look at your favorite recipes and see how you might adapt them to items that are in the storage pantry. Try to take a balanced approach to meal planning and storage. The following ratios are an example of foods that would contribute to a balanced diet:

> PROTEIN: 13 percent of your food supply. This category includes legumes, meat, peanut butter, and assorted nuts.
> GRAINS: 40 percent of your food supply. This would include cereals like oatmeal, as well as pasta, rice, and breads.
> VEGETABLES: 20 percent of your food supply. This would include carrots, peas, green beans, corn, and other vegetables.
> DAIRY: 12 percent of your food supply. This would include milk, yogurt, and cheeses.
> FRUITS: 15 percent of your food supply. This would include canned peaches, berries, and other fruits, including tomatoes.

These ratios are only a guideline and apply to a full day, so you may find that more cereal and fruit are eaten at breakfast, while proteins and vegetables make up the rest of the day's meals.

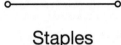

Staples

Your long-term food storage plan begins with the fundamentals, including grains, beans, fats, sweeteners, dairy items, and basic baking ingredients.

At the most basic level, every person needs about one pound of "dry matter" every day to survive. Dry matter refers to foods such as legumes, grains, sugar, pasta, dried vegetables, or rice. This matter represents calories, the stuff that is needed to produce energy in the body. A pound of dry matter represents about 1,600 calories, the low end of energy needed for the average adult. Of course, a consistent diet of dry matter would be very dull, and over the course of a few months the body would begin to suffer from the lack of protein, fresh greens, and essential vitamins. Still, it is a good starting point to keep in mind as you make decisions about what to store.

Some people do keep an emergency pantry that contains only these essentials—whole grains, dried beans, oils, and sweeteners. The problem is that these foods require you to cook in a way that may not be compatible with your current lifestyle. You need to have a basic understanding of cooking and baking techniques as well as a high tolerance for boring meals. If you decide to make these staples the center of your food pantry, take the time to learn to use them in your everyday meals.

Grains

If you don't already know how to bake your own bread, this is the time to learn! I consider homemade bread one of the most essential, and comforting, aspects of the self-sufficient lifestyle. That's why baking flours and whole grains are integral ingredients of my emergency pantry. We bake a lot, so there are pre-ground white and whole wheat flours on hand at all times. Flours have a limited shelf life, particularly the whole wheat flour, so we rotate them through our pantry all the time. We also store a variety of whole grains, including whole kernel wheat for grinding into fresh flour.

Corn, rice, and oats are also essential in our plan, and I always keep some quinoa and millet on hand. There are a number of grains to choose from, so experiment with them before deciding what you want to add to your storage pantry.

Baking Supplies

All that flour won't be very useful without having the basic ingredients for baking on hand. It only takes a few ingredients to create a wide range of baked options, from muffins and simple quick breads to yeast breads, cakes, and pies. Besides yeast, baking powder, soda, and salt, I would also add a few important baking spices like vanilla, cocoa powder, cinnamon, and nutmeg.

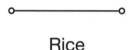

Rice

We love brown rice, but because it contains natural oils, it has a shorter shelf life than white rice does. We keep both in our pantry but make sure our brown rice is always used within three months or so and reserve the white rice for long-term storage. Rice is not only good for cooking; it can be ground into a delicious light flour for baking.

We both grew up with wild rice, so we keep that in storage, too. Wild rice is technically not rice at all, but a grain, one of the most nutritious available. It adds fiber and texture when combined with white rice and is a good source of minerals. Unlike brown rice, wild rice keeps for years.

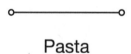

Pasta

All dried pastas keep well; easily for two years or more. Keep your favorite varieties of shapes and flavors in the pantry. In addition to elbow macaroni, spaghetti, and spirals, we also keep orzo and couscous.

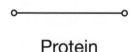

Protein

Protein in the basic pantry list includes a number of shelf-stable dried items. There is a very good variety of protein options that keep for a long time.

Canned meats include tuna and other seafood options, as well as canned chicken and other pre-cooked meats.

Dried legumes are at the center of the protein stash, with black beans, pinto beans, lentils, navy beans, and split peas among the many options. Served with rice, they are the perfect supply of protein.

Nuts, peanuts, and peanut butter are also good sources of protein. Many people think of them primarily as a high protein snack, but there are a number of creative ways to incorporate them into your cooking. We use almonds in vegetable stir fry and tacos and use peanuts as a basis for our chili. Dehydrated peanut butter powder is very shelf-stable and is good for baking. It can also be reconstituted with a bit of oil and water to make a spread.

Dehydrated eggs are great for long-term storage and can be adapted for use in any recipe that calls for eggs. Reconstituted, they make very good scrambled eggs, quiches, or omelets.

Textured vegetable protein (TVP) is made from soybeans and serves as a good replacement for ground beef in sauces, tacos, or chili. It comes in a wide range of flavors, from beef and chicken to pepperoni, sausage, and taco. TVP is reconstituted at about a 1:1 ratio.

Make Your Own Peanut Butter

Toast one pound of raw peanuts lightly in a dry skillet over low heat. Remove from skillet and cool slightly, then grind the peanuts in a grain mill or juicer. When ground to the consistency you prefer, add a couple of tablespoons of honey and blend thoroughly. Fresh peanut butter should be stored in the refrigerator.

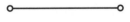

Fat

Fats are not only an essential part of the human diet, they are one of the most important ingredients in making things look and taste good! Because an opened container of oil oxidizes quickly, we store our oil in small sealed containers. Oil is best kept in cool conditions and should be rotated through your pantry every few months.

○————————○

Dairy

Dry dairy products include a wide range of options. Dry milk is an essential staple, but there are also butter and cheese powders, as well as buttermilk and sour cream options. And don't forget chocolate milk!

○————————○

Sweeteners

When you are cooking meals out of an emergency pantry, keeping a sufficient calorie intake is always a key concern. Sweeteners help to deliver the carbohydrates required for energy and allow you to bake tasty breads and desserts that are decidedly comforting. Sugars are quite stable as long as they are properly stored. Honey is exceptionally so, having a shelf life of approximately forever. And don't forget molasses and maple syrup for variety. Though not as durable as sugar and honey, they can add flavor to your staples.

○————————○

Seeds for Sprouting

These little beauties call for a category of their own. Legumes and seeds that have been sprouted carry all the goodness that you can get from fresh produce, packed with essential enzymes, vitamins, and minerals. And best of all, they capture the fresh flavor of greens that is so lacking in the basic stores of the staples pantry. They will sit, quietly dormant, until you are ready to unleash them. This category includes both seeds and legumes that are created specifically for sprouting.

Alfalfa, broccoli, radish, clover, chia, and sunflower sprouts provide a fresh delicacy that replaces spring greens. Mung, lentil, pinto, adzuki, and soy beans provide the durable freshness that fits perfectly in a stir fry.

Make sure you buy untreated seeds that have never been sealed in airtight containers. Seeds need to breathe to be able to sprout.

○————————○

Extras

These are the items that give you the opportunity to turn simple ingredients into flavorful meals. Store bouillon cubes and soup bases as well as pre-mixed soup seasonings. Add your favorite seasonings to the pantry, too, but stick to the ones you know and like best.

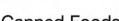

Canned Foods

Once you have established the list of pantry staples that work for your family, it is time to add canned fruits, vegetables, and other foods to your list. Most canned foods keep for eighteen months to two years, so they should be a regular part of your rotation plan.

A One-Year Emergency Pantry

To feed a family of four for a full year, a pantry that consists entirely of staple ingredients will look something like this:

500 pounds of whole grain wheat for grinding	12 pounds of honey
100 pounds of flour	12 pounds molasses or maple syrup
100 pounds of cornmeal	12 pounds jam
100 pounds of oats	12 pounds of sprouting seeds
50 pounds of quinoa	40 quarts of vegetable oil
50 pounds of millet	240 pounds dry milk
200 pounds of rice	48 cans evaporated milk
100 pounds of pasta	4 pounds baking powder
120 pounds dried beans	4 pounds baking soda
20 pounds lentils	2 pounds yeast
20 pounds split peas	20 pounds salt
40 pounds soy beans	2 gallons vinegar
16 pounds peanut butter	20 pounds dry soup mix
1½ gallons dehydrated eggs	A variety of spices and seasonings
50 pounds TVP	
160 pounds sugar	

o———————o

Fruits and Vegetables

Fruits and vegetables are an essential part of a daily diet. If you are a gardener, you may have a ready supply of fresh or preserved produce.

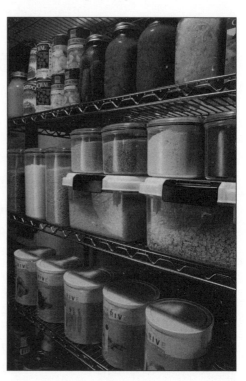

An enormous array of commercially canned vegetables, fruits, tomatoes, and beans are readily available and easy to store. Choose your family's favorites and add to your stockpile each week. We keep canned applesauce, peaches, pears, pineapple, mandarin oranges, cherries, and some of our favorite berries at all times and rotate them over a twelve- to eighteen-month period.

Among our favorite canned vegetables are artichokes, sweet corn, peas, green beans, mushrooms, tomatoes, olives, and onions. Don't forget those beautiful orange vegetables—pumpkin, squash, and yams are all great out of the can.

o———————o

Other Canned Foods

Because beans are such a big part of our diet, I keep plenty of canned legumes on hand. We love garbanzo beans in salads and pasta dishes. We store pinto and black beans in whole bean cans and also use canned refried beans. Kidney beans and a variety of white beans are in the pantry for adding to soup or chili.

Our pantry would not be complete without some commercial pasta sauces and salsas, along with pickles, mayonnaise, barbecue sauces, and mustards. Though these might be considered a luxury to some, to us they are part of everyday meals, and as such have a place on our shelves all the time.

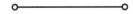

Dehydrated Foods

Fruits and Vegetables

Dehydrated fruits and vegetables are a great part of the emergency food pantry. Because of the way they are processed, they actually retain more of their nutrients than either of their canned or frozen counterparts. Most single-ingredient dried foods are processed without salt, a real plus for my family. A serving of dehydrated green beans contains 0 mg of sodium versus a serving of canned green beans, which contains 380 mg.

Fruits and vegetables can be dried or freeze-dried. Dried foods are a common part of many people's diets—jerky, raisins, fruit roll-ups, potato flakes, and seasoned soup mixes are just a few of the dried foods we encounter in the grocery store. Drying can be done at home by applying low heat to your chosen food. Drying removes up to 98 percent of the moisture of the food, leaving you with compact, lighter weight storage. Stored properly, dried foods can keep for one to three years in your pantry.

Freeze-drying is a more sophisticated method of drying that allows the food to retain its nutrients, along with its flavor, color, and shape. Even lighter in weight than dried foods, a #10 can of freeze-dried vegetables contains forty to fifty servings, yet weighs less than three pounds. The shelf life of freeze-dried foods is generally considerably longer than standard dried foods, as much as twenty-five years for an unopened can.

I keep dehydrated vegetables on hand to use as flavorings in cooking, or as a base for soups or stews. Dried onion flakes, chile, and bell peppers, carrots, celery, mushrooms, spinach, broccoli, and garlic are among the dried vegetables in our pantry, along with some pre-mixed soup blends. We also keep potato flakes for making mashed potatoes and potato soup.

Dried fruits make great wholesome snacks. Dried apples, apricots, bananas, dates, as well as prunes and raisins, can be kept in the snack section of your pantry. Reconstituted fruit can be used just as you would any canned or frozen fruit.

Other Dehydrated Foods

There are a number of handy convenience foods that would also fall into the category of dehydrated food. These include boxed puddings, baking mixes, and gravy powders, as well as Ramen noodles, macaroni and cheese, and other all-in-one boxed supper blends. Consider your family's taste to determine which of these belong on your own shelves.

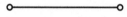

Pet Food

Our animals are part of the family, and their foods have a place in our emergency pantry. An extra bag of kibble is always there, along with a couple of cases of canned food and treats.

It is important that pets have access to clean, fresh water. Small dogs or cats should have about a pint of water a day, while larger dogs may need up to half a gallon a day.

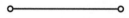

Non-food Supplies

While you could probably get by without all the luxuries of your current home kitchen, there are a handful of items that really must go into your staples supply. Keep a supply of bleach, basic cleaning supplies, and toiletries such as toothpaste, feminine hygiene products, toilet paper, and shaving gear. We also keep a supply of disposable wet wipes and hand sanitizer for personal and clean-up use.

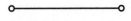

First Aid

Ready-made first aid kits are fine, but we prefer to make up a complete first aid kit of our own. It contains enough of the basics to get us through just about anything. Our kit includes:

Burn ointment	Matches	Petroleum jelly
Triple antibiotic cream	Thermometer	Prescription medicines
Hydrogen Peroxide	Cold medicine	Rubbing Alcohol
Adhesive bandages	Antacids	Epsom Salt
Small splints	Antibiotics	Elastic bandages
Gauze	Anti-diarrheal	Hot and cold packs
First aid tape	medicine	Heavy string
Small scissors	Syrup of ipecac	Sunscreen
Tweezers	Antihistamines	Aloe cream for
Sterile cotton balls and	Laxatives	sunburns
swabs	Multi-Vitamins	

Personalized Meal Planning

In order to have the most cost-efficient and useful food pantry, you will want your inventory to be filled with only the items that your family likes to eat. (Of course, if their diet currently consists of McDonald's and steak, this might be a little tricky.)

If there are staples that your family does not currently eat, but that you would like to make part of your emergency inventory, begin to work those foods into your everyday meals. Don't go out and buy a twenty-pound bag of TVP and hope for the best. Instead, try replacing ground beef with TVP at your next taco night. Add beans to a pot of vegetable soup or make quesadillas with refried beans before investing in a case of beans. Do a "meatless Wednesday" every week to try different recipes and get your family used to new ingredients. Once you feel comfortable that an ingredient has been accepted, add the recipe to your list.

How much do you need?

Start by choosing seven recipes that you know your family enjoys. Write out the list of ingredients and multiply the quantity of each ingredient by the number of times you would like to be able to serve it.

For example, my family likes Mexican-style foods, so a simple meal straight out of my pantry may be a casserole consisting of one cup of uncooked rice and two cans of chili-spiced black beans, along with one cup of corn and one cup of chopped tomatoes. If I want to be able to serve this meal once a week for twelve weeks, I will need to multiply all the ingredients in this recipe by twelve.

In this example, I need twelve cups of rice. Since I won't be buying my rice by the cupful, I next need to take my list and convert it to quantities that my ingredients are actually sold in. In the case of the rice, there are about two and a half cups of uncooked rice in a one-pound bag of rice. Since I need to store twelve cups of uncooked rice for this recipe, I will need about five pounds (twelve divided by two and a half). Convert the rest of your ingredients in the same way to determine how much to buy.

Ingredient	Quantity	Amount Needed to Serve 12 times	Conversion
Uncooked Rice	1 cup	1 x 12 = 12 cups	12/2.5 = 4.8 pounds
Black beans	2–15 oz cans	2 x 12 = 24 cans	24 cans
Corn	1–15 oz can	1 x 12 = 12 cans	12 cans
Diced tomatoes	1–8 ounce can	1 x 12 = 12 cans	12 cans
Chili powder	1 tablespoon	1 x 12 = 12 tablespoons	12/4 = 3 ounces
Cumin	1 teaspoon	1 x 12 = 12 teaspoons	12/13 = about 1 ounce
Salt	1 teaspoon	1 x 12 = 12 teaspoons	12/5 = 2.4 ounces

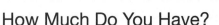

How Much Do You Have?

If you were talking about your financial investments, you would know exactly how much you have, right? Treat your food account in the same manner. It is important to know how much you have, how much you use, and how much you need in order to manage your food pantry effectively.

The Food Planning Chart at the back of this book is a good template for taking an inventory of what you currently have. Use it as a guide to think about what you want in each category and remove items that do not fit into your plan. Use the blank lines in each section to note items that are not listed on the Planning Chart. Record the item, the quantity, and, if applicable, the size of the container.

Now is a great time to clean out your cupboards! Take a look at expiration dates and throw out anything that is past its prime. If you have food items that you know you won't ever use, set them aside and take them down to the local food bank. Make a mental note about the kinds of impulse purchases that didn't work out and resolve not to fall victim to that kind of shopping.

How Much Should You Buy?

Once your inventory is complete, record in the next column how much of each item you would like to have on hand, based on your recipe planning. To determine your shopping list, in the Planning Chart, subtract the Amount on Hand from the Amount Needed, and place that figure in the Amount to Buy column.

I recommend that you make a plan for three months of back-up food. Your three-month plan should be well-balanced and include a combination of family favorites, staples, baking goods, and non-food items. If you create a solid three-month plan, expanding it to six months or one year is simply a matter of adding the same items you have established.

○────────────○

Shopping for Your Food Pantry

If you plan wisely, every penny you put into your food pantry will be like money in the bank. But like most savings accounts, it doesn't get there all at once. It is not necessary, and may not even be desirable, to run out and stock your pantry in one shopping trip. In addition to the fact that it may take time to accustom your family to new ingredients, it also takes time to develop a knack for managing and rotating foods. Plan for a certain amount of trial and error as you begin.

○────────────○

The Grocery Store

You may think that all this planning is beyond the reach of your budget. It's not! The worst thing you can do is avoid beginning until you feel you have extra money to spend on your pantry project. Your grocery store is a good place to start. Watch for specials and take advantage of them. Rather than procrastinating, try dedicating as little as $10 a week to your grocery budget to get started. You will have the pleasure of seeing your shelves fill up in surprisingly short order.

A $10 Per Week Savings Plan

Week One
5 pounds of white rice
1 pound of beans
1 48-ounce bottle of vegetable oil

Week Two
5 pounds of flour
1 pound of honey
2-3 packs of yeast
26 ounce of iodized salt

Week Three
25-ounce box of dry milk
Sprouting seeds

Week 4
12 cans of assorted canned fruits, tomatoes, and vegetables

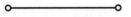

Shopper's Clubs

If you belong to a shopper's club and can buy larger quantities in bulk, the unit price will certainly be lower than normal grocery store shopping. Begin by buying extra quantities of the items you are certain you will use. Just make sure to balance your purchases so your pantry is not a lopsided storage unit for mismatched foods.

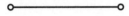

Food Co-ops

Food co-ops are another great option. Co-ops are member-organized stores or buying clubs that provide food items at the best prices to their members. They are a great source for bulk grains, beans, and spices, as well as fresh local produce. But before you bring home a big sack of bulk ingredients, know what your storage plan for it is. Plastic bags are okay for short-term storage, but for protection against pests and humidity, you will want to use airtight storage containers.

Emergency Resource Stores

There are companies that sell whole systems of dry and dehydrated food storage ingredients. These are generally packed into one-gallon cans, known as #10 cans. They are well-sealed and definitely ready for storage, with shelf lives extending to twenty-five years. You may find that you are comforted by the presence of a balanced selection of crucial items such as rice, grains, dried vegetables, and powdered milk.

The Shelf Reliance Company is a good resource for this kind of food. They have a comprehensive inventory of storage foods, systems, and meal planning guides.

Farmer's Markets

Almost every small town in America has a farmer's market—a place for local farmers and growers to come and offer fresh local produce and handmade products. During the height of growing season, these markets are a delight, but they can also help you to provide for your off-season pantry as well. Bushels of tomatoes, fruits, and other produce are readily available at a good price. If you like to

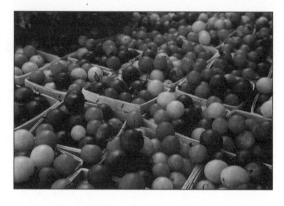

be in control of your food source and are up for the task of preserving your own food, the farmer's market is an excellent resource.

Buying from farmers encourages the local farming and gardening economy and reduces the energy footprint of the food you eat. The locavore movement, which encourages people to rely on local sources of food, makes a strong case for relying on food produced within 100 miles of where you live. Fresher, riper food, lower food costs, and less reliance on the fossil fuels required to get the food to you are some reasons to go this route. But even more important to some is the taste; a tomato allowed to ripen naturally on the vine is far tastier than one picked in another country

and ripened on its journey to your grocery store. Local food also encourages greater appreciation for the effort that goes into growing produce and meat for your table, particularly if you have the opportunity to visit the local farms they come from.

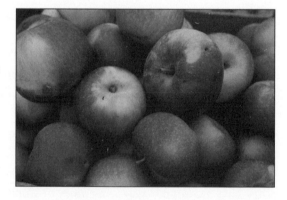

Community Supported Agriculture

Another powerful movement that allows you to tap into local resources for fresh produce and other farm products is Community Supported

Agriculture (CSA). There are many variations of this concept, from buying "shares" in a local farmer's crop to community gardens that require some shared labor in exchange for a portion of the harvest.

The CSA concept has grown exponentially in recent years, with some estimating that there are now over a million of these programs across the country. If you look into your local CSA, consider these things before deciding to join:

- Is the food portioned out equally among members or do you have a say in what you get?
- Are you willing to eat produce that is straight out of the garden? Some people find the idea romantic, but then are turned off by dirty, hard-to-wash greens food items they don't know how to cook.
- Are you willing to take the same risk that farmers take when they plant their crops? If you purchased shares and conditions turn against the harvest, your stake may be at risk, too.

Bartering for Food

It can be very liberating to know that you can get what you want without using money. Bartering is as simple as trading what you want for what someone else needs. Start by figuring out what you have that may be of value to someone else. Maybe you grow terrific tomatoes but are wishing you had fresh eggs. If you can find a chicken farmer who doesn't spend a lot of time in his garden, you may have a deal. He may even be willing to trade you some of that wonderful manure he is producing in exchange for a portion of next year's crop.

Maybe you make great pies and your friend makes wonderful baked beans. Or maybe you want to help with someone's canning in exchange for some of the final product. Once you start thinking in this way, the possibilities are endless.

When you find a like-minded person who is willing to trade goods or services, hammer out the details. If you are just swapping those tomatoes for the eggs, a handshake may suffice. But for many trades, it is best to put these details in writing, particularly if you are trading for services.

Designate what you will do and what you will receive. Set how much time will be allocated to it and name a deadline to complete services.

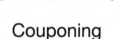

Couponing

Couponing has been raised to an art form in recent years, with frugal shoppers making the most of bargains available through a combination of manufacturer's coupons and local store deals. So how do you get started?

Find the coupons The first step in couponing, of course, is the coupon. You can find coupons in newspapers, magazines, in the grocery store aisles, online, on previously purchased packaging, and direct from the manufacturer. You will find a wide variety of products available at a discount, but be partial. It's only a bargain if you really need it. Choose items that your family genuinely uses on a regular basis.

Organize As you collect your coupons, devise a strategy for organizing and keeping them handy. Your system may be as simple as separate envelopes sorted by category, or as complicated as a three-ring binder sorted by aisle and expiration date. Make sure to clean out your system regularly; you don't want to carry around a bunch of expired coupons.

Use Them Make the most out of your coupons by frequenting grocery stores that offer double and triple coupon days. Take a look at your grocery store flyer to see if you can match their sales to your coupons and increase your savings even further. Dedicated couponers have many other ways of maximizing their savings, so if you enjoy this type of shopping, do your research.

Building Your Pantry

Location, Location, Location

While you can tuck three days' worth of food just about anywhere, when you make the commitment to store three or more months' worth of food, location matters. You want the location to be cool and dry, away from direct sunlight. But almost as important, you want it be located in an area that is easily accessible, where you can take inventory, unpack new items, and grab needed ingredients easily. Walk around your home and evaluate available spaces.

The Basement

Cooler temperatures usually prevail in the basement, making it a good candidate for your pantry. Take note of any moisture problems. If your basement suffers from leakage or tends to be damp, it may not be the best location. Make sure you have an area that is positioned away from the furnace, hot water heater, or washer and dryer.

Root Cellar

Some older houses have a root cellar—a space dug underground specifically designed for food storage. Cellars generally have dirt floors and have a fairly stable temperature and steady humidity year-round. Although they may not be practical for storing canned goods and other items that require a dry environment, they are great for extending the life of fresh fruits and vegetables. If you are lucky enough to have a root cellar, use it for storing a winter's worth of potatoes, carrots, cabbages, and other hardy produce.

The Garage

It is tempting to place storage shelves in the garage, where extra space may be readily available. Be aware, though, that there are not many geographical locations where the garage is a good choice. The temperature of the pantry should not be subject to wide temperature swings, and it is a rare location that doesn't have freezing winter temperatures or scorching summer heat. The humidity at our home in Virginia works decidedly against the garage. After evaluating all our options, we did choose to use our garage for our pantry, but did so by building a well-insulated 8 x 13 foot space in the back of our garage to create a room that could be climate-controlled. Additional shelving in the main garage space holds emergency non-food items like toilet paper and paper towels as well as pet food and some water.

If you live in a northern climate that has consistently freezing temperatures, the garage can be a good place to store grains because the freezing condition can kill bugs that make their home in grain. Just make sure that they are well packaged—a garage is also an inviting retreat for rodents seeking a little respite from colder outside conditions. All it would take to make their retreat perfect would be a free supply of readily accessible grain!

The Attic

There are a couple of things that make the attic a less-than-attractive option for food storage. The first is that most attics are un-insulated, making them very hot in the summer. In the winter, they are favored by squirrels and other rodents. The second thing is that most attics are difficult to reach, often only by a ceiling hatch or ladder. This makes the prospect of going back and forth to fetch items or unpack new inventory daunting.

Some older homes do have half-story spaces that may not be desirable as bedrooms but are accessible by stairs and heated and cooled with the rest of the house. Spaces like this may be a good choice for your pantry.

The Spare Bedroom

Some of the best food pantries I have seen were set in spare bedrooms that were dedicated just for that specific use. Lined with shelving units as neat as a library's stacks, these rooms are the ideal location for a food pantry.

Laundry Rooms, Utility Closets, Porches, and Breezeways

As soon as we saw the laundry room in our new home, we knew we could greatly enhance the efficiency of its space. We immediately built additional shelves above the washer and dryer to hold cleaning supplies and paper goods, and tore out the decorative, though wasteful, cabinets above the utility sink in favor of sensible shelving. Because this room is right off the kitchen, it is ideal for often-used food ingredients.

It is amazing the space you can find if you only look. Friends of ours had a semi-heated back porch that held a spare freezer and nothing else. With the addition of floor-to-ceiling shelves, they converted this space into not only an efficient storage facility, but into a veritable showcase for the power of the food pantry. Guests entering through this back entrance cannot help but stop and admire the neat rows of cans, bins, and tubs, all labeled and dated.

Closets

The average bedroom closet can store a lot of food when built out to maximize the placement of pantry shelves. Plan shelf height based on the specification of your storage bins. If you use five gallon buckets, place them on the floor, and position the next shelf high enough for easy clearance. Place successively lighter goods on higher shelves.

The Kitchen

I am blessed with two pantries in my kitchen. The first, which we refer to as the baking pantry, holds all our flour, grains, sweeteners, oils, and baking supplies, with the top shelves used for assorted bread pans, cookie sheets, and the like. The second pantry, which was originally a broom closet, was re-fitted with shelves that perfectly fit our cans and other often-used ingredients. I try to keep three or four of my most-used canned goods, pastas, staples, and snacks in this closet, replenishing it as needed from our larger storage space.

The reality is that most kitchens, even small ones, would benefit tremendously from simple organization. Uniformly sized containers help make inefficient space hold twice what it otherwise would. Likewise, supplemental wire utility shelving can be used to double the storage capability of conventional shelves.

Small Spaces

What if there are no cupboards, pantries, or spare walls for fancy shelving? There is one great unused "closet" in every household that you might not have thought of. That place is under the bed. With an empty 60 x 80 inch space under a queen-size bed, there is room for an entire pantry under there. If you want to add even more space, consider putting your bed on risers. Risers can add five inches of storage space.

There are a number of standard underbed plastic bins or wheeled carts available for storage. Of course, #10 cans fit nicely under most beds, too. There is even an under-the-bed rotation system made specifically for cans.

Treat your underbed pantry as you would any other shelf. Devise a rotation system that allows for ready access to foods. One method is to fill your pantry on the left and withdraw from the right. Or if you are using a bed that is up against a wall, start at the top and withdraw from the bottom.

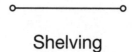

Shelving

Now that you have settled on the location for your Food Pantry, it is time to organize it! There is a wide variety of shelving systems and organizational accessories, and they come with a wide array of price tags.

Plan Your Space

Before you go shopping for shelving, consider your space. Do you have just one flat wall available for storage, or do you have the luxury of room for multiple shelves?

If you have the space, consider placing shelves so that they are accessible from the front and the back. This will make rotation and replenishment of your stock much easier.

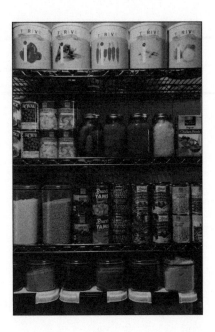

Converted Closets

Do you have a spare closet just ready and waiting to be used? If so, consider how you will utilize it. You can purchase flexible shelving systems with adjustable shelf heights, or you can build stationary shelves. If you take the latter approach, choose and measure your containers so you know just how high each shelf should be. If you have enough depth, consider buying can rotation accessories to allow for horizontal storage of your cans.

Shelf Capacity

The capacity of your shelving will depend on how you organize it.

- Make sure you know what the recommended weight capacity is for the shelves you choose. Commercial shelving has capacity ratings that can range from several hundred pounds to seven thousand pounds. Don't immediately assume that metal shelves are stronger than plastic. Review the manufacturer's specifications when deciding.
- Match containers to your shelf height to achieve maximum capacity.
- Place larger, heavier items on bottom shelves and lighter objects on top.
- If you already have standard shelves, look for accessories to help you organize. Can organizers for horizontal storage on standard shelves are

available in deluxe heavy-duty plastic versions as well as inexpensive cardboard styles.

- If you have the budget, consider buying a rotation shelf system. They come in a range of widths and are customizable for the can sizes you plan to store. The Shelf Reliance Company has a large assortment of these shelves.
- If you have room, put heavy items such as grains and flour in large containers on the floor of your storage space. If your floor is concrete, add a moisture barrier before putting down containers. An old pallet or even a piece of carpet works fine.

Containers

Decide what size containers you plan to use based on how long it will take you to use the food.

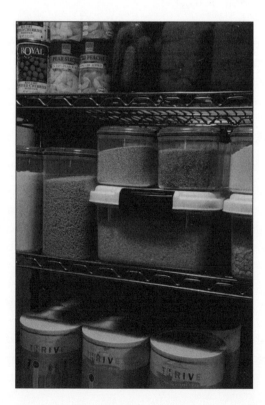

Standard Fruit and Vegetable Cans

These range from small tuna cans to the large cans of fruits and vegetables. I store many of my fruits and vegetables, as well as cooked legumes and other prepared food, in these. It gives my pantry plenty of variety, allows me to open only what I want, and it is easy to add to my pantry a little at a time. You can choose from small cans that contain only one to two servings up to the large twenty-nine-ounce cans that contain up to six servings. Try to stick to cans that are appropriate to your recipes and don't be tempted by oversized sale offerings. Canned foods should be used within eighteen to twenty-four months.

#10 cans

Great for items you use a lot, as well as foods that are very stable, even when open. A #10 can generally holds around four to five pounds of grains, sugar, or dried beans. Sealed #10 cans have a long shelf life—over eight years or more. Once opened and exposed to the air, you should plan on using the contents within a year or two. Every ingredient is a little different, so check out the manufacturer's recommendations for shelf life.

A #10 can of cornmeal holding about four pounds is about how much I would be willing to have open at any one time. Cornmeal is quite stable and an opened can will be okay to use for about a year. If I thought I could use enough corn in a year to warrant the purchase of a five-gallon bucket, it would certainly save me money to purchase it that way. But I prefer to store several #10 cans of cornmeal, knowing that most of my store is well-sealed, with only what I need exposed to the air. Otherwise, we may be eating a lot more cornbread than I had intended!

Food Grade Buckets

Anything that has a very long shelf life, and that you use in sufficient quantities, can be purchased and stored in five-gallon buckets. A five-gallon bucket of white flour, for example, contains about thirty pounds, and has a shelf life of about six months after it has been opened. I bake often enough to make that worth my while. Many grains and beans have an opened shelf life of one year or more. If those fit nicely into your food plan, then go ahead and store them in five-gallon buckets.

Mylar Bags

These food-grade metalized bags are used for lining food storage containers. Mylar bags create an oxygen, moisture, and light barrier to help keep long-term food storage fresh. They are available in sizes ranging from sandwich-size bags to five gallon buckets, and can be sealed using an ordinary household iron.

Oxygen Absorbers

Oxygen is the enemy when it comes to food freshness because it creates a good environment for pests, aerobic pathogens, and molds. Oxygen absorbers can help reduce the oxygen level inside your container, keeping your food fresher for a longer period of time. It is important that they be used in airtight containers; any air leakage will negate the effectiveness. These small packets generally contain iron powder and are suitable for use with dried goods that contain less than 10 percent of moisture. Follow the manufacturer's directions for use.

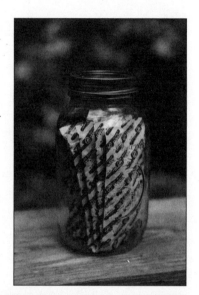

Using Oxygen Absorbers

Oxygen absorbers begin absorbing oxygen the moment they are exposed to air, so don't open your packages until you are ready to use them. Remove only the number you need and immediately place the remaining absorbers in a glass jar with a tight lid.

Airtight Containers

Once your food is opened, the original container may not be the appropriate choice for its storage. Any food will be kept fresher and longer by placing it in a container that seals out exposure to the air. Choose airtight containers with good snap-on lids. Don't assume any lid will do; if you live with high humidity like we do, the conventional plastic lids that come on your cans don't do a good enough job of keeping out humidity.

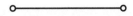

Establishing Your Pantry

You have chosen your location, your beautiful new shelving, and a working plan for the foods, sizes, and storage containers you plan to use. So what goes into storage first? I suggest you follow this order for filling your pantry:

Water

Before you buy one single can of food, get your water in place. Loss of power is the number one reason that families lose access to fresh drinking water. That means that even a sudden thunderstorm may knock out your ability to use your tap water for a few days.

You should have at least a two-week supply of drinking water. Plan on one gallon per day for each member of your household. For a family of four, that is fifty-six gallons. (Don't forget some for the pets.)

Commercial water jugs range in size from one to five gallons, or you can fill any food-grade plastic container from your own tap. Large water storage systems are also available, ranging from the standard fifty-five-gallon barrel all the way to home storage units with capacity for several hundred gallons.

Emergency Supplies

Make sure your first aid kits, batteries, flashlights, fuel, and other crucial supplies are stocked and ready.

Three-Day Supply

If you haven't already done so, make sure your pantry is ready for a three-day emergency, one that could include loss of power. This is the most common emergency that befalls the average family, so before you start long-term storage, make sure this is ready.

Balance Your Pantry

You are now ready to embark on your three-month supply! Some experts suggest that you start your pantry by adding one food group at a time. While that sounds like an orderly approach, I prefer knowing that whatever money I have invested is on a path to creating a balanced pantry.

Think about a typical morning. How does your family start the day? In most families, this is the most well-established routine of the day. Do you need coffee, tea, milk, sugar, fruit, and cereal? Establish a list of breakfast items that you would need for several weeks and work on having all of them on hand. I learned this the hard way when I started building my pantry. I got excited about the supply of beans and grains I was gathering, but hadn't gotten around to buying dried milk. When a hurricane stranded us for a few days, I quickly saw the hole in my plan—there wasn't even enough milk for our coffee! Simple as it sounds, this small omission created more than a little inconvenience—black coffee and dry cereal was a serious disruption in my family's normal routine!

Keep an eye on your inventory list and try to add to each category—a couple of #10 cans of grain, a case of canned fruits and vegetables, a few pounds of beans, some dry milk. Stick with your recipes and evaluate the usefulness of your pantry every week. If you are overloaded with grains, but lacking in baking ingredients and seasonings, you may find yourself with a very limited emergency menu.

Learn to Use New Foods

Now that you have begun collecting family favorites, it is time to stretch your cooking skills, along with your family's food repertoire. Learn to bake bread, cook a good pot of beans, sprout seeds, and make your own yogurt. Experiment with using reconstituted dairy and egg products and replacing meat with other ingredients. As your family becomes comfortable with certain foods, add those to your pantry.

Add the Fun

Long-term storage doesn't have to all be serious! Boxed cake mixes, dried pudding, tortilla chips, powdered drink mixes, popcorn, your favorite crackers . . . these all have a place in your storage pantry. If your family is like mine, it won't be hard to rotate these through your pantry, but read the manufacturer's label for shelf life.

Non-food Items

Some non-food items are pretty crucial, so I make sure a good supply of toilet paper and wet wipes are part of my standard three-month supply. But after you are well along with your food purchases, consider what other items to add. You may want paper plates, extra cleaning supplies, and basic personal products such as deodorant, shaving creams, and soaps. Keep a list of the family's favorites; these products are often featured on sale and in coupons.

5

The Specifics of Food Storage

Every item in your pantry needs to be stored in the following three conditions to maintain optimum quality: cool, dry, and dark. High temperatures, humid or wet conditions, and exposure to light are the primary reasons for spoiled food. In addition, food must be kept safe from bugs and rodents. Keep these factors in mind when storing any food products. The following are specific recommendations for each food group.

Long-term Storage of Whole Grains, Beans, and White Rice

Whole grains, dried beans, and white rice are very durable, but they must be stored in a cool, dry location. Temperatures of 50–60°F are ideal for ensuring maximum longevity. Overheating or wide temperature swings will shorten their life. Likewise, humidity causes challenges. Any time moisture is present, there is a danger for molds and bacteria to grow.

Bulk foods used for long-term storage should be carefully sealed to keep them safe from pests and rodents. To store a large quantity of dried bulk foods, choose food-grade five-gallon buckets with gasket lids. Line each bucket with a Mylar bag. Place one 500cc oxygen absorber in the bottom of the bag. Fill the bag about half way, shaking the bucket to settle the food.

Add another oxygen absorber and then fill the bucket, leaving about an inch of space on top. Place another oxygen absorber on top.

Pull the bag up as high as you can, settling the food into the bucket. Use a hot iron to seal the Mylar bag. Place a board on the edge of the bucket, lay the bag top straight, and start sealing the bag from left to right, making sure to squeeze out excess air before finishing the seal. Fold the bag down and place the gasket lid on the bucket.

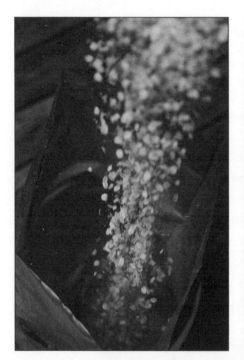
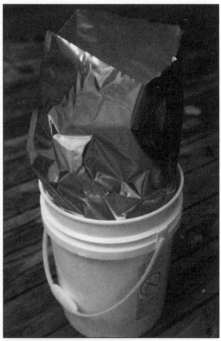
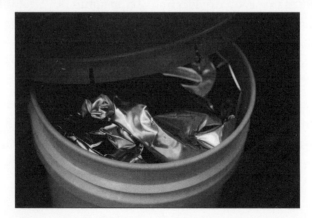

How to Store Flour

For long-term storage, whole grains are definitely the way to go. Flours tend to be more fragile and most will keep for less than a year. Whole grain flours in particular do not keep as long because the germ portion of the whole grain causes the flour to become rancid over time.

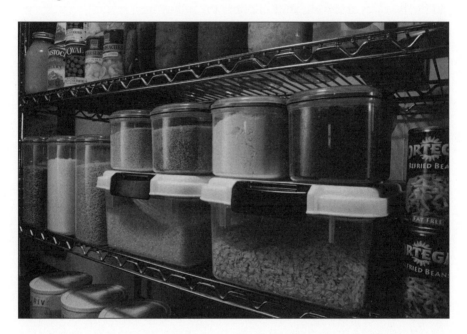

If you are rotating flour every couple of months, remove it from the paper container it came in and place it in a sealed container to keep it fresh and protect it from pests. To store white or corn flour for longer than a few months, pack it into re-sealable plastic bags, squeezing out as much air as you can before sealing. Place bags in the freezer for a few days to kill any living organisms. Store bags inside a five-gallon bucket using the sealing method above.

Pasta is more durable than flour and can keep up to eight or ten years in an airtight container, safe from moisture.

○———————○

How to Store Fats and Oils

Like all items placed in storage, oils need to be protected from heat, light, and oxygen. Over time, any oil will begin to oxidize, turning rancid. Oil becomes rancid long before we can detect it, so unlike with other foods, a simple sniff and taste test will not tell you whether your oil is still good. To do the best job of storing your oil, note the following:

- Choose lighter vegetable oils for storage, rather than the more flavorful dark olive oils and specialty oils, which tend to have a shorter shelf life. Coconut oil is also a good choice; it tends to be somewhat more stable and can be kept for at least two years.
- Find the coolest place in your house to store oils. Even unopened containers generally only have a shelf life of about a year, so check the manufacturer's date stamp.
- After opening, place oil in a glass container with a good seal. If you can use darkened glass, all the better. Refrigerate opened oil; unrefrigerated oil can start turning rancid within weeks. Don't worry if your oil becomes cloudy in the refrigerator; it is still perfectly good.
- Because of oil's relatively short shelf life, any oil you keep in your pantry should be carefully rotated. Buy small containers so you only have to open what you can use within a month or so.
- Shortening is another good choice for storage. An unopened can of shortening can keep up to ten years. Shortening, butter, and peanut butter powders can also be stored by up to five years or more in sealed containers, but should be used within one year of opening.

○———————○

How to Store Yeast

Keep yeast in its original packaging. Storing yeast in a cool location is best; yeast kept in a cool pantry will be good for up to two years, while frozen yeast can be kept much longer. Refrigerate all unopened yeast if you can.

Because yeast is a living organism, it must be alive to work its magic. To test the viability of your yeast, place one and a half teaspoons of yeast, along with one teaspoon of sugar into one-fourth cup of warm water. Set aside for about ten minutes. The yeast mixture should bubble up during that time, doubling to about one-half cup. If it doesn't, it won't have the strength to raise your bread adequately.

o———————o

How to Store Dry Milk

Dry milk is an important part of the food pantry. Besides being used for drinking, it is an integral ingredient in baking recipes. In addition to calcium, milk also delivers needed vitamins A and D. It is important to keep milk fresh, particularly to preserve the vitamins which can be lost through exposure to light.

Milk is highly absorbent so dry milk packaged in cardboard should be immediately placed in a glass container with a tight fitting lid to prevent it from absorbing moisture and odors. This is important even if your milk is for short-term use. Keep it in a darkened pantry or in the refrigerator.

For long-term storage, buy #10 cans that are factory sealed, but remember, an airtight seal does not immunize the milk from moist or high temperature conditions. Milk requires the same care regardless of the container. If you want to pack your own larger containers of milk, you may store them in large buckets using the method outlined for grains.

o———————o

How to Store Sugar, Honey, and other Sweeteners

Sugar is a very durable foodstuff and requires nothing more than a dry container to stay good for a long time. All types of sugar, whether white, brown, or powdered, are highly susceptible to moisture and easily conduct odors, so place your bagged sugar into an airtight container. If sugar is exposed to moisture, it will get hard and lumpy, but it will still be okay for use. Use the method outlined for grains to store large quantities of sugar in buckets.

Honey is the original long-term sweetener (containers of edible honey have been found in ancient tombs!). Honey keeps very well indefinitely. Buy only pure filtered honey and store it in glass containers in your pantry. If honey crystallizes, just place the container in hot water until it melts.

Molasses and maple syrup are great to have around for baking and breakfast. Molasses is my favorite sweetener for baking; I love the rich darkness it adds to breads and cookies. You should keep both of these syrups in a cool, dark place and use within two years.

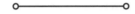

How to Store Salt

Salt keeps indefinitely and has many uses, so keep a good quantity of it in your food storage. It is an integral ingredient, not only for cooking, but for preserving and drying foods.

Iodized salt, which has a small amount of iodine added, is generally processed with anti-caking ingredients. Iodine is a crucial nutrient not found in many foods other than seafood, so it's good to add iodized salt to your meals.

Kosher salt is a coarse salt that is produced without caking agents. It dissolves quickly and can be used for brining or curing meats.

Sea salt can be purchased finely ground or in coarse crystals. We love the flavor of these natural salts, which tend to carry along the mineral flavors from where they were produced.

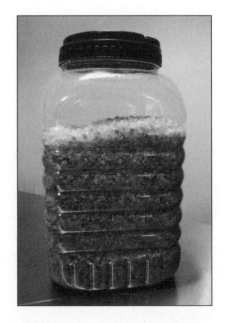

Pickling salt is a finely ground salt that is produced without added iodine, used specifically for brining and canning vegetables, pickles, and sauerkraut.

Curing salt is a combination of salt and sodium nitrate. It is used to preserve and cure meats, as well as in sausage making. You will generally find it in a pink color with a small amount of red dye added.

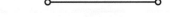

How to Store Dehydrated Foods

Pre-packed dehydrated foods should be stored in a cool, dry location. Once opened, they should become a regular part of your food rotation and are best used within a year or so. Commercially dried or freeze-dried foods have very low moisture content, and an opened can may be susceptible to humidity. If you live in a humid area, consider transferring opened dried fruits and vegetables to glass storage containers.

Home-dried foods generally have higher moisture content than commercially prepared foods. Store your dried foods in airtight containers. I prefer to use home-dried fruits and vegetables within six months, but depending on the moisture content and your own storage conditions, they may last longer. Homemade jerky is best used within a month or so.

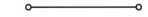

How to Store Canned Foods

Canned goods will form a large portion of your pantry and are easy to store. Commercially canned products should be stored in a cool, dry place. A temperature of 50–75°F is ideal, with relatively low humidity. Don't be tempted to bargain shop for dented cans, especially those you plan to put into storage. A small dent may be okay, but deep dents are just inviting trouble.

Canned goods generally have a "best if used by . . ." date stamped on their labels. This is a voluntary date that is placed on the can by the manufacturer, and is meant to indicate how long the food will be at its absolute best. It is not an actual expiration date. Canned food that is past the date on the can is most likely still perfectly fine. In fact, it will probably continue to be good for use for many months after. You can use the manufacturer's guideline to gauge the age of your food, but the best way to find out whether it is edible is to open it, check its appearance, and smell it.

Canned foods will last for several years under good storage conditions. Canned fruits, tomatoes, and tomato-based sauces will generally keep their freshness and color for twelve to eighteen months. Canned vegetables generally will keep their freshness and color for about two years. Canned legumes, canned soups, stews, and meats have an even longer shelf life of two to five years.

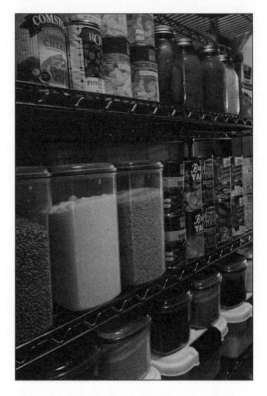

The "best by" date is irrelevant if the can has swelled or is leaking. Discard any cans that are heavily rusted, have been frozen, or smell "off" when opened.

I rotate my home-canned foods a bit faster than my commercial cans. After all, I grew and canned them myself so I want to use them at their freshest. High acid foods such as fruits and tomatoes should be used within a year or so, while low acid foods will last a bit longer. You may notice some rust on the metal rings, but as long as the seal is okay, the food should be fine.

○────────────○

Shelf Life of Foods

"Sealed" refers to hermetically sealed containers. These are estimates, and will vary based on storage conditions. Check the manufacturer's dates for specific information.

For commercial products, check the manufacturer's "best by" date, and use that as your "sealed" date.

	SEALED	**OPEN**
PROTEINS		
Canned ham	2–5 years	3–4 days in refrigerator
Freeze-dried meats	25 years	1 year
Commercially made jerky	2 years	1 year
Home-dried jerky	1–2 months	1–2 months
Hard/dry sausage	6 weeks in pantry	3 weeks in refrigerator
Dried eggs	12–15 months	Refrigerate after opening. Use within 7 to 10 days. Use reconstituted egg mix immediately or refrigerate and use within 1 hour.
Canned tuna	18 months	3–4 days in refrigerator
Other canned meats	18 months	3–4 days in refrigerator
LEGUMES		
Dried beans	30 years	5 years
Instant dried beans	30 years	1 year
TVP	10 years	1 year
Peanuts		
Peanut butter, natural	2 years from manufacturer's date	2–3 months
Peanut butter, emulsified	2 years from manufacturer's date	18 months
Peanut butter powder	4 years	1 year
GRAINS AND FLOUR		
Wheat	10–12 years	2 years
Dry corn	10–12 years	3 years

Continued on next page

Millet	10–12 years	4 years
Flax	10–12 years	4 years
Barley	8 years	18 months
Quinoa	20 years	1 year
Rolled oats	8 years	1 year
Whole wheat flour	2 years	6 months
White flour	4 years	1 year
Spelt flour	5 years	8–12 months
Flaxseed flour		2–3 months
White rice	10 years	1 year
Brown and wild rice	1–2 years	6 months
Pasta	8 years	3 years
NUTS		
In the shell	9 months	6 months
Shelled nuts	2 years	18 months
FRUITS AND VEGETABLES		
Low-acid canned goods, such as soups, vegetables, stews	2–5 years	3–4 days in refrigerator
High–acid canned goods, such as fruits, tomatoes and vinegar–based items	12–18 months	5–7 days in refrigerator
Home–canned foods	1 year	3–4 days in refrigerator
Dehydrated fruit	25 years	12–18 months
Dehydrated vegetables	25 years	1–2 years
BAKING SUPPLIES		
Yeast	2 years	4 months
Honey	10 years	2 years
White sugar	30 years	2 years
Brown sugar	10 years	1 year

Molasses	2 years	6 months
Baking powder, baking soda, and salt	30 years	2 years
Vinegar	2 years	1 year
Spices and seasonings	2 years	2 years
Boullion	5 years	2 years
OILS		
Cooking oils	6 months	3–6 months
Shortening	2 years from manufactured date	1 year
Shortening powder	10 years	1 year
DAIRY PRODUCTS		
Dry milk	25 years	2 years
Sour cream powder	10 years	1 year
Cheese, dried	15 years	6 months
Butter powder	5 years	9 months
OTHER		
Seeds for sprouting		4 years

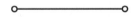

Rotation

The "Store What You Eat and Eat What You Store" family pantry is a living, breathing organism. It is designed to be used every day, not just in an emergency. Because, for the most part, you are stockpiling foods that are a standard part of your family's diet, you should have an easy time keeping foods fresh and using them before their expiration date.

Always remember FIFO—first in, first out. Develop a system. You can keep older items front and center on your shelf, and fill your shelves from the rear when you add new foods. Or you can store from left to right, always using from the left and adding on the right. Food rotation shelving helps you create an almost foolproof system for your canned goods, helping you keep track of which food to consume first.

I have a "ready rack" in my kitchen—a shelf that contains some of everything I keep in long-term storage. This allows me to "go shopping" in my large pantry to stock the small one, and gives me the chance to look through my inventory, make adjustments, and note things that need to be replenished.

Check your manufacturer's label for the freshness date. Don't just assume that the date you purchased it means it is the freshest. For bulk foods, or other foods that have no manufacturer's date on your food, add a label with your purchase date. Make sure to label and date all home canned and preserved foods.

Check your inventory list on a regular basis and note any products that are not being used as quickly as planned. If you have purchased something that your family doesn't like, don't wait until it expires to remove it from your pantry. Take it down to the local community food pantry so someone else can make use of it.

Remember to rotate grains and other bulk storage items. Never add new product to the top of your existing storage container. Take the time to pour out whatever is left in the bucket, place the new product in the container, and then pour the older product on top. If you have more than the container can hold, pour the leftovers into a spare container for immediate use.

6

Cooking Off the Grid

One of the most common emergencies people face is loss of power. If you have a generator or a gas cook stove, you may feel adequately prepared. But other situations do occur, such as earthquakes and severe storms, when you may not have access to your home gas lines.

For people who rely entirely on electricity and have no other back-up options for generating power, figuring out how to cook food can become a problem. You should understand your options for alternatives, whether for a short-term emergency cooking plan or long-term solutions.

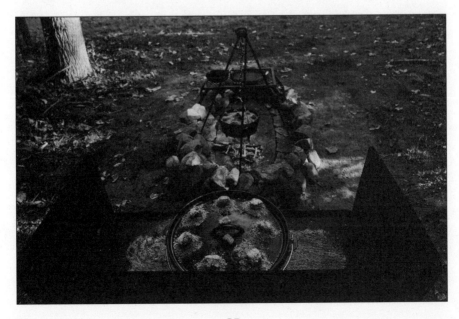

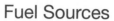

Fuel Sources

Butane Canister

This fuel is most common for its use in lighters, but can be purchased in a can for camping or emergency use. This fuel should be used with a stove designed specifically for burning butane. Outside of camping stores, canisters of butane can be hard to find. For short-term emergencies, a butane stove and several canisters can be kept in your storage pantry.

Canned Heat Cell Fuel

Like butane, this fuel is designed for short-term use. Small heat cell fuel cans, such as Sterno, are used with stoves designed especially for use with them. This is a lightweight, easy-to-store single burner solution for emergencies. The fuel lights up quickly and can be re-lit again and again. It is very stable, so it does not require special storage considerations and has an indefinite shelf life. Each can of fuel provides about five hours of cooking time. It's a sensible fuel option to have for your three-day food supply.

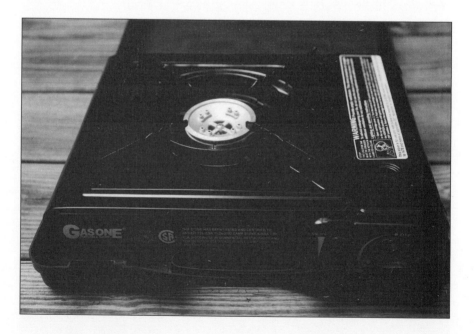

Propane

Propane is a great option for emergency stovetop cooking. Because propane is so readily available for home grilling use, it is usually easy to purchase and replenish. It is available in small one-pound canisters for emergency use, or in large tanks like the type typically used in gas grills.

If you wish to buy standard grill tanks, consider whether you want the option to refill them at any propane filling station. Some propane tank purveyors consider themselves "tank swap" suppliers, and have mechanisms that can only be filled by them.

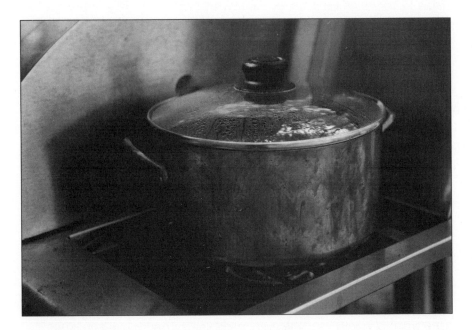

Usage

Propane tanks are generally measured in pounds. A typical grilling tank is about thirty pounds and holds about seven gallons of fuel.

To calculate how much burn time your tank will provide, first find out how much the empty tank weighs. This number should be engraved on the tank with the letters "TW." Weigh the tank on your bathroom scale and subtract the empty tank weight from the weight of the canister. The resulting number is the amount of fuel in your tank.

Every pound of propane provides about 21,600 BTUs, but the amount of burn time depends on your stove. Look for the manufacturer's published BTU output to calculate usage for your specific stove or grill. You can find the manufacturer's BTU output labeled on the stove or in the instruction manual that was included with your stove. BTU efficiency ranges from 1,000 to 20,000 depending on the type of stove and heat required.

Multiply the pounds of fuel you have in your tank by 21,600. For example, ten pounds of fuel will provide about 216,000 BTUs. Next, check the manufacturer's BTU output for your stove. This number refers to the burn capacity for one hour. If using a 10,000 BTU grill, ten pounds of fuel should provide about twenty-one hours of cooking time. Of course, these are just estimates. Actual cooking time depends on a number of factors, but this will help give you a rough idea of your needs.

Storage

Make sure you check that the valve is tight before storing your tank. Because propane is explosive, as well as toxic, store it outside, away from the house. Propane can be stored indefinitely, but there are generally laws regulating how much you can keep on hand, so check your local rulings. It is not safe to bring propane tanks into the house, so use stoves and grills outside only.

Wood and Charcoal

If firewood is readily available, it's a good source for heat and cooking. Dry hardwood is the best choice; soft woods such as pine and poplar tend to burn too quickly. A wood fire requires about forty-five minutes for coals to reach the proper temperature. Wood coals tend to be inconsistent in size and do not last as long as charcoal briquettes, so you have to tend the fire more carefully when doing anything but the most basic simmering.

I have found that charcoal briquettes are much easier to use for controlling and maintaining heat. Good charcoal briquettes are a more consistent size than campfire coals and they burn longer and more evenly.

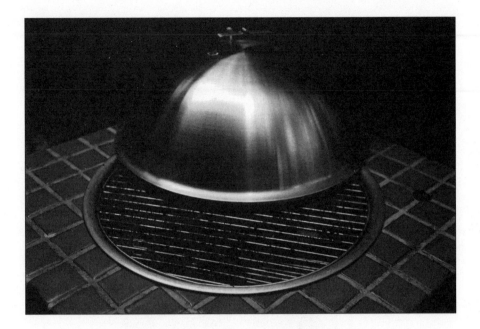

They are easier to move around, too, allowing you to adjust your heat quickly and easily.

Usage

Wood and charcoal are not space-saving fuels. To cook for your family for an entire month, you may need 100–200 pounds to provide the needed heat for cooking three meals a day.

Dry wood has about 7,000 BTUs per pound. The drier your wood is and the lower its resin content, the more efficient it will be in producing heat. A good, well-seasoned oak will provide about 24 million BTUs per cord, compared to only 16 million BTUs if you used it freshly cut. Compare that to dry white pine, which only provides about 14 million BTUs. Plan to use 100–300 pounds of wood to cook for one entire month. Wood usually requires a supply of kindling to get the fire started, so make sure to keep a supply of small combustible pieces readily available.

Charcoal has about 9,000 BTUs per pound. To rely on charcoal for all your cooking needs for an entire month, you can expect to use about 120–150 pounds. Use a charcoal chimney and paper to start and prepare your charcoals for cooking.

Storage

Cut and split hardwood into twelve- to eighteen-inch lengths. Stack wood in a location with plenty of wind and sun so that it has the chance to become dry and well-seasoned. The length of time it takes to season wood depends on weather conditions and seasonality, as well as the wood variety. Winter-cut wood has less sap, so it seasons more easily than summer-cut wood. In general, freshly cut wood should be dried for four to six months before use. Keep stacked and seasoned wood lightly covered so that the outside surface stays dry. If wood has to remain uncovered, keep it bark-side up and cut side down, if possible. The drier the wood, the higher its usable energy for burning.

Keep charcoal briquettes in a dry, re-sealable container to keep them from getting damp and absorbing too much moisture.

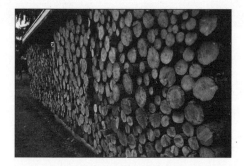

Building an Outdoor Fire Pit

To build a fire pit for cooking or staying warm, choose a location with plenty of open space around it. Avoid overhanging branches and roofs that could catch fire, as well as wood floor surfaces that might be damaged by falling coals. Dig a shallow hole that is about three feet wide and one foot deep. Line the hole with large flat rocks. Cold earth tends to suck the heat out of a fire and the rocks will make the pit easier to pre-heat. Make sure it is level—uneven surfaces not only lead to uneven cooking, but with all that hot coal and simmering food, they can be dangerous.

Even a small breeze can play havoc with your cooking temperatures, so carry some kind of shield in your gear to keep out the wind. Any kind of makeshift breeze block will help you keep your fire burning nicely and prevent ashes from blowing into your food when you lift the lid.

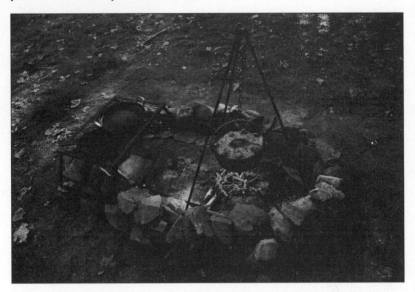

Build your fire of wood or charcoal on top of the rock surface. You can place a cast iron Dutch oven right onto the coals. To use a regular pot or skillet, find a grate to fit over the hole to use for grilling and simmering. Keep a fireplace shovel handy for moving embers and cleaning out ashes. And don't forget the marshmallows.

Cooking with a Dutch Oven

For me, when it comes to cooking off the grid, there is nothing that compares to the Dutch oven. The Dutch oven is a fryer-broiler-stewer-roaster-steamer-baking oven all in one. It is designed to keep moisture in and retain and circulate heat directly around your food.

Off-the-grid cooking often means outdoor cooking—and that brings with it a number of factors that have to be considered. Wind, air temperature, humidity, location, and your cooking surface all play a part in how you will generate and maintain your heat. A little wind can gobble up your coals faster than you had planned, while high humidity can slow the burning down, and a shady location or cold ground surface can lower your temperature by 25°F or more.

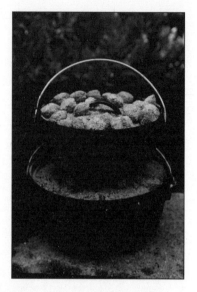

Calculating Heat

Because the Dutch oven is such a versatile cooking unit, it only makes sense that there are a number of ways to heat and cook with it. That's why I tend to calculate my coal needs myself, based on a few basic rules.

A single charcoal briquette generates around 15°F. That means to maintain a temperature of about 350°F, you would need to use approximately twenty-four coals. This is handy to know, but not entirely reliable because it doesn't factor in oven size or other conditions. It is just a good starting point.

It is always best to be a little conservative when starting out. An overly hot oven can burn your food. It's easier to build the heat than it is to cool down a hot Dutch oven.

○────────────○

Dutch Oven Cooking Methods

Laying coals for different types of cooking is a matter of ratios. The first number always refers to the coals you will put on top of your oven. The second number is the number of coals you will put on the bottom. For example, 4:1 means four times as many coals on the top of the oven as on the bottom. One the other hand, 1:4 means that there would be four times as many coals on the bottom as on the top.

Boiling and Frying

These are the most basic methods for cooking with your Dutch oven because all the heat is underneath. The temperature is kept high for the entire cooking process. This is the one time that you would use an entire spread of charcoal as your heat source. There is no need to produce a huge mound of charcoal—too much heat can actually harm the oven. Just lay down a single layer of coals directly under the oven.

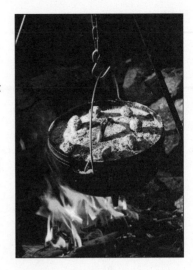

Simmering and Stewing

We use this method for soups, stews, and other recipes that require slow simmering. The primary heat source is underneath the oven, with a few coals on top to keep everything warm. A ratio of 1:4 is about right for simmering.

Stewing and simmering does not call for sophisticated calculations, just a bit of common sense. A few coals on top will help the entire oven to stay warm. Start with eight coals on the bottom and two on the lid for a twelve-inch Dutch oven, and adjust your temperature up and down by adding or removing coals.

Roasting

Meats are generally cooked using even heat. For roasting, we use a 1:1 ratio. That means that the heat source is evenly distributed on the top and the bottom of the oven.

To start, take your oven size and double it to get the total number of coals needed. For example, a twelve-inch oven would require twenty-four coals. Place twelve coals on top and twelve on the bottom to maintain a 350°F temperature.

Baking

While roasting is somewhat forgiving, baked recipes call for a little more precision. Baking requires more heat on top of the oven than on the bottom to keep the bottom from burning and to ensure even cooking on top. For baking, we use something closer to a 3:1 ratio. A quick way to calculate the right number of coals is the three up/three down rule.

Step 1	Start with the diameter of your Dutch oven.	12-inch oven
Step 2	For your top heat, add 3 to the diameter of your oven.	15 top coals
Step 3	For your bottom heat, subtract 3 from the diameter of your oven	9 bottom coals

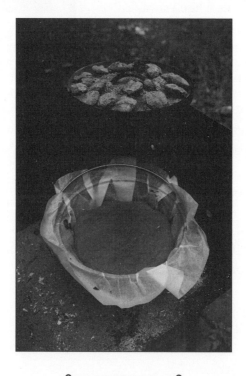

Cooking with a Solar Oven

This is the gentlest and most environmentally friendly method of cooking; nothing but the sun is needed to produce great meals. The solar oven comes in a number of variations, but it is essentially nothing more than a box that concentrates and traps the heat of the sun. The food inside is gently cooked at a temperature of around 325°F. To cook your food, all you do is place it inside the oven, position the oven directly under the sun, and wait. Think of it as a natural crock pot.

The solar oven works very well when the sun is in full force, so it is designed for use during the day. The only tending needed is to check and adjust its position every couple of hours to make sure that it is getting the full force of the sun. Because your food won't burn, there is no need to stir or fuss with it during its cooking time. Since no smoke is produced and the gentle heat never reaches dangerous temperatures, the solar oven can be left unattended.

A bright sun is the only requirement for cooking, but even on the sunniest day, cooking times will be affected by factors such as outside temperatures, wind, and elevation, so it may require a bit of experimentation to learn the time needed to cook your food. Smaller batches work best—small cuts of meat rather than large roasts, sliced potatoes instead of whole ones. A small pot of rice will cook in approximately four hours, a simple chili or stew four or five hours, a small roast in about six hours. The solar oven will bake basic breads or cookies, but it will not brown them like a conventional oven.

I like the Sport Solar Oven from the Solar Oven Society, a non-profit organization dedicated to promoting solar cooking both in the United States as well as in third-world countries that lack consistent energy sources. It is reasonably priced, lightweight, and easy to pack for camping trips.

○———————○

Natural Refrigeration—The Zeer Pot

This clever natural cooling system relies on evaporative cooling and is widely used in locations where refrigeration is unavailable. Evaporative cooling works like this: a liquid evaporates into the air, cooling the objects that it is in contact with. A Zeer pot is made by placing one pot inside another pot, separating them with a layer of wet sand. The smaller inner pot is where you store your food. As the water evaporates from the sand, it draws the warmth out of the smaller pot. Zeer pots are designed for dry and arid conditions; they do not work well in climates with high humidity.

To make a Zeer pot for yourself, use a large porous (unglazed) earthenware pot. The smaller pot that fits inside should be glazed to prevent the moisture from the wet sand to seep into it. Place a thick layer of sand between the two pots, wetting it thoroughly. Cover with a wet towel.

A Zeer pot can keep foods cooler than ambient conditions do, often cool enough to extend the life of meats, cheeses, vegetables, or milk for several days. To keep the cooling process going, you can set the large pot in shallow water so it can continue to absorb moisture into the sand. Or you can wet the sand between the pots twice a day.

7

Using Your Storage Pantry

There is a wonderland of good cooking awaiting you in your pantry if you just know how to use it. Grains can be turned into beautiful breads, dried milk into yogurt, and humble seeds can powerhouse sprouts. Take the time to add one new ingredient to your pantry one at a time, and learn how to cook with each.

Whole Grains

Storing whole grains seems like a sensible idea in theory, but now that you have those bags of wheat and corn, what do you do with them? It may seem daunting to get used to making these foodstuffs an everyday part of your diet, but if you have no desire to learn about them, there is not much point in storing them.

This recipe is an easy way to get started. Make a batch of the dry ingredients and you will have a ready-made side dish waiting in your pantry. Try other grains such as millet or quinoa using this recipe. If you would like to try making your

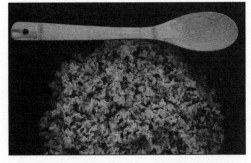

own multi-grain mix, make sure to cook grains that have similar cooking times together.

Herbed Rice Mix

  3 pounds long grain rice
  2 cups dried celery flakes
  ⅔ cup dried minced onion
  ½ cup dried parsley flakes
  2 tablespoons dried chives
  1 tablespoon dried tarragon
  3 to 4 teaspoons salt
  2 teaspoons pepper

Mix together all ingredients and store in a large glass jar with a tight-fitting lid.

To prepare rice, bring two and a half cups of water to a boil. Add one cup of rice along with two tablespoons of olive oil. Reduce heat and simmer for twenty minutes. Fluff with a fork and serve.

COOKING WHOLE GRAINS			
1 cup grain	**Required liquid**	**Cooking time**	**Yield**
Amaranth	6 cups	20 minutes	2 ½ cups
Barley	3 cups	60 minutes	3 ½ cups
Buckwheat	2 cups	20 minutes	4 cups
Bulgar	2 cups	10 minutes	3 cups
Millet	2 ½ cups	30 minutes	4 cups
Oats, steel cut	4 cups	30 minutes	3 cups
Quinoa	2 cups	15 minutes	3 cups
Brown Rice	2 ½ cups	30-45 minutes	3 cups
White Rice	2 ½ cups	20 minutes	2 ½ cups
Wheat Berries*	4 cups	60 minutes	3 cups
Wild Rice	3 cups	45 minutes	3 ½ cups

*Soak overnight before cooking.

Grinding, Cracking, and Flaking Grains

There are grain mills available in a range of models and prices. Hand grain mills require a little more manpower than an electric mill, but they are capable of producing good fine flour. For most bread, a finely textured flour is desirable because it exposes more of the grain's gluten. This helps you produce lighter, more finely textured bread. Of course, a bit of coarse flour makes for an interesting texture, so go ahead and mix in some coarse with the fine. (I would limit coarse flour to about a half cup for one two-pound loaf.)

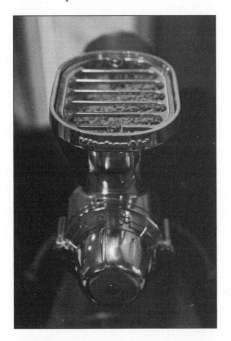 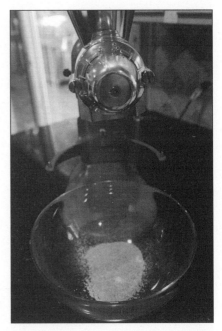

Keep only a few pounds of whole grain open in your pantry, and store in a cold place if possible. A freezer is ideal, but a tightly sealed container in a cool pantry is fine. Grind only as much flour as you need; fresh flour loses its nutrients rapidly and the oils can turn the flour rancid in only a few days. If you have extra flour, store it in the freezer.

Making Oatmeal

You can make your own flaked grain. Freshly flaked oatmeal is a revelation— the chewy texture is so much better than store-bought oatmeal that was flaked who knows how long ago, and contains all the nutrients that generally start disappearing soon after grinding.

Start with clean hulled oat groats and grind through the flaker to your desired consistency. Grain flakers usually have settings for regular flake, quick cook flake, or cracked grain. Other grains can also be flaked or cracked to make interesting multi-grain hot cereals. Freshly flaked oatmeal cooks in about ten minutes.

Making Bulgur

Bulgur is wheat that has been parboiled and then dried. It is not cracked wheat, as some people assume, although you can crack the parboiled wheat if you wish. The advantage of having bulgur on hand is that it cooks very quickly and is great as a side dish or a salad. Bulgur is generally made of Durham or white wheat without chaff, although any wheat can be processed using this method.

To make your own bulgur, rinse your whole wheat and drain. Place the clean wheat in a pot and cover with fresh water. Cook until tender, about thirty-five to forty minutes. Drain any excess water and spread the cooked wheat on a cookie sheet, and place in a warm 200°F oven to dry. Then cool the wheat.

If you wish to crack your wheat, make sure it is very dry. The drier the wheat, the easier it will be to crack. Crack the dried wheat in your food mill on a coarse setting. Store in an airtight container.

Making Grits

Grits are traditionally made with white corn, although some people swear by yellow corn grits. The secret to grits is the texture; you want as fine a texture as possible for cooking grits. Start by cracking your corn at the coarsest setting. A manual grinder can be used but corn is remarkably tough, so plan on using some elbow grease. Once your corn is cracked, return it for another round of grinding. Repeat this process three or four more times. Finally, sift corn through a fine screen.

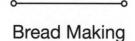

Bread Making

Even if you never needed your emergency supply of food, it is worth the effort to learn your way around whole grains, milling, and baking your own bread. Homemade bread is the food of the gods, and your ability to make great breads starting with the whole grain is a skill worth having.

The basis of bread is gluten. Gluten is the protein in the bread that traps the gases given off by the yeast, raising the bread and giving it its nice elastic texture. But not every grain contains gluten. Gluten is found in wheat, as well as in spelt and Kamut (khorasan wheat). These grains need to form the majority of your bread flour.

For a recipe calling for four cups of flour, at least three cups should be high gluten flour. The other cup of flour can be anything you like; rice flour, oats, millet, quinoa, rye, etc. It is fun to experiment to make your own multi-grain loaf.

Making Perfect Whole Grain Bread

Freshly ground whole wheat flour is just the beginning of great bread. The recipe that follows meets all the requirements for taste, nutrition, and texture, whether you are already a fan of whole grain bread or just introducing it to a finicky family.

The reality is, there are many ways to get a beautiful loaf of bread, and this is only one of them. Bread requires just a few ingredients—flour, yeast, liquid, and salt, along with just a bit of sweetener to encourage yeast production. Everything else is optional.

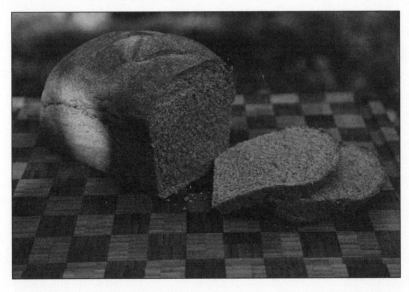

Big, Beautiful Whole Wheat Bread

2½ teaspoons active dry yeast

½ cup lukewarm water

½ cup lukewarm milk

½ cup orange juice

5 tablespoons olive oil

1½ teaspoons salt

3 tablespoons sugar

¼ cup dry milk

¾ cup instant mashed potato flakes

3¾ cups whole wheat flour

Proofing

The magical ingredient in bread is yeast. Yeast converts fermentable sugars into gas, causing the dough to rise. I grew up proofing my yeast—essentially double-checking it to confirm that it was still active. I still consider it a good practice, especially for yeast that has been stored for a while. Yeast does not die suddenly, but rather goes flat over time, so old yeast may raise your bread, but not as energetically as it should.

To proof your yeast, start with lukewarm water (about 75–80°F). When you run the water on your wrist, it will feel neither hot nor cold. This is important because yeast will be killed at temperatures of 100°F or higher. If you are new to bread making, use a thermometer to learn what 80°F feels like. Place one half cup of warm water in a small bowl and add active dry yeast. Throw in a big pinch of sugar for good measure, to give your yeast something to feast on. This process takes about ten or fifteen minutes. I enjoy seeing the bubbles form on the surface of the water; it gives me the assurance that my yeast is active and ready to go.

Dry Ingredients

While your yeast is proofing, get out a large bowl and add whole wheat flour along with dry potato flakes, dry milk, sugar, and salt. Make sure your wheat flour is finely ground to ensure good rising. The potato is a great starch for your yeast to feed on and helps to create a moist, tender loaf. The milk gives the bread sweetness, along with a little extra nutrition. Sugar and salt add flavor, but make sure you put in the correct amount. Too much sugar can inhibit the gluten, while too much salt will inhibit your yeast. The correct ratio of salt to flour will help control yeast development. If it is not present, your yeast may overproduce and cause your bread to collapse.

Liquids

Pour in warm milk, orange juice, and olive oil into your proofed yeast. The milk should be just slightly warm, and it will help brown the loaf. The orange juice can go in straight out of the refrigerator. It is an optional ingredient, but goes a long way to neutralize the slight bitterness of whole wheat that children may not like. Olive oil (or butter, if you prefer) adds enough fat to ensure a tender crumb and it keeps the bread fresh a bit longer.

Start stirring, incorporating the liquid into the flour until your dough is thick and sticky. Because flour absorbs moisture, the amount of flour you actually need is a bit of a guessing game. (Real bakers weigh their flour for this reason; this way they know exactly how much they need.) If your weather is humid, you may need less flour, if it's dry, you may need a bit more.

Kneading

When the dough has formed a ball and is solid enough to be handled, pick it up and set it on a lightly floured surface. Knead it gently, rotating it one fourth turn as you go, until it forms a solid ball that has the supple weight of clay. Don't add flour as you knead; that tends to create a tougher, heavier loaf.

Rising

Place your dough in a lightly oiled bowl, cover, and set it aside until it has risen to approximately double its original size. For whole wheat, this usually takes ninety minutes or more. When it is ready, punch it down and return to the kneading surface, quickly shaping it into a smooth log. Place it in a lightly oiled loaf pan. Cover again and let rise until it is no more than an inch over the rim of the pan. This process usually takes an hour or more.

Baking

Preheat your oven to 350°F. Never place your bread in a cold oven, always start baking when the oven has reached the proper temperature. Bake bread for about ten minutes and then add a loose tent of foil to prevent over browning of the surface. Bake another thirty to thirty-five minutes.

Remove from the pan immediately and cool on a rack. For a soft crust, coat loaf with butter or oil.

○———————○

Cooking with Beans

Beans are an integral part of our diet and for good reason. Not only are they versatile, but most beans can be cooked whole, ground into flour, and even sprouted. They are a great source of protein, particularly when combined with rice to form a complete protein.

Basic Beans

Cooking beans in the following way reduces the gassiness that some people associate with eating them and also gives you nice whole beans that are not broken or mushy.

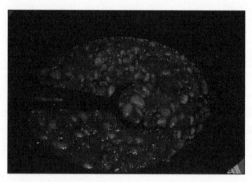

    1 cup dried beans, rinsed and cleaned (pinto, black, kidney, Great Northern, navy, or cannellini)
    Water
    Salt

    Wash beans and make sure there are no small stones or other debris present. Place in a large bowl and cover with boiling water. Soak overnight.

    The next morning, drain beans and rinse. Place back in pot, cover with fresh water, and bring to a boil. Once beans are boiling, continue to cook for about five minutes. Remove from heat, skim foam, drain, and rinse.

    Place beans in fresh water, bring to a boil, then turn heat to low and simmer for about one hour. (Kidney beans usually require a little more time so add about fifteen minutes when cooking these. Navy beans may be ready in forty-five to fifty minutes.) For quicker beans, cook in a pressure cooker for about eight minutes. Or if you have all day, place on low in a crock pot for six to eight hours.

When beans have reached your desired texture, drain them and season. Add salt only after cooking; beans cooked with salt tend to be a little tough. One cup of dried beans will yield 2½ cups or so. If you don't need your whole batch of beans at one time, place rinsed beans in zipper freezer bags and store leftovers in freezer until next time.

Grinding Beans into Flour

A number of bean types can be ground into flour for use in soups, as thickeners, or even in baking. Bean flour adds extra nutrition and fiber to a wide range of recipes. Black bean flour can be used in chocolate cake or dark breads, or reconstituted into an easy black bean soup. White bean flours, such as the type made of soy, navy, or garbanzo beans, can be used as thickeners and in dips and baked goods.

Small beans such as lentils may be made into flour in one step. Working in small batches, just blend beans until they are pulverized and powdery. Remove from the blender and continue making small batches, until you have as much as you need. (One pound of beans makes about two cups of flour.) With larger beans, you may need a two-step process; the first to crack the beans, the second to grind them into flour.

Baking

Bean flour adds punch to everything from bread and chocolate cake to pancakes and biscuits. Use any of your normal recipes, but substitute 25 percent of your regular flour with bean flour. Because bean flour has no gluten, you may add only a little to yeast breads. In quick bread and griddle recipes, like the pancake recipe below, bean flour can do all the work.

Bean Flour Pancakes

¾ cup garbanzo bean flour
½ teaspoon salt
1 teaspoon baking powder
1 tablespoon oil

½ cup water

1 egg

Beat together all ingredients to make a smooth batter. Pour ¼ cup onto a lightly oiled preheated griddle. Serve with butter and syrup or applesauce.

Thickening

Blend ¼ cup of bean flour with enough water to make a paste. Stir slowly into soups, gravies, or stews, and cook until thickened, as desired.

Refried Beans

You can reconstitute bean flour to make refried beans. Just whisk together ¾ cup of bean flour with 1 cup of water. Cook on low heat for five minutes or so. Instant beans!

Condensed Soup

Use about 6 tablespoons of any white bean flour. Whisk it into 2 cups of water, and add 4 teaspoons of chicken bouillon granules for flavor. Simmer until thick. Makes a great substitute for any recipes calling for condensed cream soup.

o———————o

Soups and Stocks

I am a huge fan of soup. Not only is it easy to make, it stretches easily into a satisfying meal with the addition of a hearty loaf of bread. It also is endlessly versatile, allowing you to create satisfying recipes with whatever ingredients are on hand.

While your pantry may be stocked with bouillon cubes, canned stock, and bases, I have included recipes here for homemade stock. Leftover meats and vegetable scraps make a wonderful base for almost any kind of soup.

Beef Stock

Olive oil

4 pounds meaty bones from the butcher

½ pound stew meat or trimming scraps

2 onions, peeled and quartered
2 carrots, peeled and cut into chunks
Celery tops or a couple of ribs
2–3 cloves garlic
Fresh parsley
2 bay leaves
8–10 peppercorns

Place bones, scraps, carrots, and onions in a large roasting pan and sprinkle all over with oil. Roast in an oven at 400°F for about forty-five minutes, turning occasionally until bones are nicely browned. Remove meat and vegetables from pan and place them in a large stock pot. De-glaze the roasting pan on top of the stove with a half cup of water. Use a spatula to scrape the browned bits from the bottom of the pan. Add this to the stock pot. Add celery, garlic, parsley, bay leaves, and peppercorns. Fill the pot with water (to within 2 inches of the top) and cover loosely with foil. Bring to a boil and then simmer on low heat for three to four hours.

Spoon excess fat from the top of the pot, remove the bones and vegetables, and strain stock into another pot through a fine mesh sieve. Let cool to room temperature and then refrigerate.

When ready to use, remove any solid fat from the top of the stock and discard. Freeze extra stock for later use.

Chicken Stock

Leftover bones and skin from a roasted chicken
2 onions, peeled and quartered
2 carrots, peeled and cut into chunks
Celery tops or a couple of ribs
Fresh parsley
2 bay leaves
8–10 peppercorns

Place the chicken carcass and all the rest of the ingredients into a large stock pot and cover with cold water. Bring to a boil and then simmer on low heat for three to four hours. Spoon excess fat from the top of the pot, remove the bones and vegetables, and strain stock into another pot through a fine mesh sieve. Let cool to room temperature and then refrigerate. When ready to use, remove any solid fat from the top of the stock and discard. Freeze extra stock for later use.

Vegetable Stock

1 large onion, quartered
2–3 carrots, cut into chunks
Celery tops or a couple of ribs
3 cloves garlic
1 leek, green and white, chopped
1 parsnip
1 tomato, chopped
4–5 sprigs of fresh thyme
1 bay leaf
1 bunch parsley
10 peppercorns

Place all the ingredients into a large stock pot and cover with cold water. Bring to a boil and then simmer on low heat for one to two hours. Remove the vegetables and strain stock into another pot through a fine mesh sieve. Let cool to room temperature and then refrigerate. Freeze extra stock for later use.

Make Your Own Dried Soup Mixes

When it comes to cooking, there are some days when inspiration just doesn't strike. I make up my own bean soup mixes for days like that, along with some inexpensive bulk versions of fancy commercial blends.

Bean Soup Mix

3 cups of assorted beans, including kidney, split peas, black beans, lentils, and white beans.

Seasoning Mix

2 teaspoons chicken bouillon granules
1 tablespoon dried minced onion
1 tablespoon dried celery
1 tablespoon dried sweet pepper flakes

1 tablespoon dried carrots

1½ teaspoons salt

1 teaspoon dried parsley flakes

½ teaspoon black pepper

½ teaspoon garlic powder

4 tablespoons brown sugar

Combine dried beans and place in a quart-size glass jar. Mix seasonings, put them into a plastic bag, and place the bag at the top of the jar. To make soup, rinse beans, cover with water, and soak overnight. Drain beans, place them in a large pot with 6 cups water, a 29-ounce can of tomatoes, and seasoning mix. Simmer two to three hours.

Lentil Barley Soup Mix

¾ cup medium pearl barley

½ cup dried lentils

2 tablespoons dried parsley flakes

¼ cup dried minced onions

¼ cup instant beef bouillon

2 tablespoons dried celery flakes

½ teaspoon dried thyme leaves

2 bay leaves

¼ teaspoon black pepper

¼ teaspoon dried minced garlic

Place all ingredients together in a quart canning jar. To make soup, add jar ingredients to large pot with 10 cups of water. Simmer one and a half to two hours.

Chicken Noodle Soup Mix

1 cup uncooked fine egg noodles

1 tablespoon instant minced onion

1 tablespoon dried carrot dices

3 tablespoons chicken bouillon granules

1 teaspoon pepper

½ teaspoon dried thyme

1 bay leaf

Combine all ingredients in a pint jar.

To prepare soup, add contents of jar to 2 quarts of boiling water. Reduce heat and simmer fifteen minutes. Stir in 3 cups cooked chicken and simmer until heated through.

Potato Soup Mix

2 cups instant mashed potatoes

1½ cups dried milk

2 tablespoons instant chicken bouillon granules

2 teaspoons dried minced onion

1 teaspoon dried parsley

¼ teaspoon black pepper

¼ teaspoon dried thyme

1½ teaspoons salt

Mix all ingredients and place in quart glass jars. To use, combine ½ cup of soup mix with 1 cup of boiling water.

Cream of Chicken Soup Mix

2 cups dry milk

¼ cup chicken bouillon granules

¾ cup cornstarch

1 teaspoon onion powder

½ teaspoon dried thyme

¼ teaspoon pepper

Mix together all ingredients and pack them into glass jar. To substitute one can of cream soup, combine 1¼ cups water and 1/3 cup soup mix in a small saucepan, whisk together, and cook over low heat until thickened.

French Onion Soup Mix

¾ cup dried minced onion

⅓ cup beef bouillon granules

¼ teaspoon celery seed

½ teaspoon dried parsley

⅛ teaspoon black pepper

½ teaspoon sugar

Blend ingredients and store in a glass jar. Use as you would commercial French onion soup mix. For dip, combine 5 tablespoons with 2 cups sour cream and let sit for at least an hour before serving. For soup, simmer 5 tablespoons of the mix with 4 cups of water.

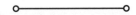

Using Dairy Products

Making Your Own Yogurt
    1 quart warm water
    1⅔ cups dry milk
    ½ cup store-bought plain yogurt with active yogurt cultures (or buy a
        yogurt starter)

If you are starting with dry milk, make a quart of liquid milk using warm water and a little more powder than you would normally use. If you are starting with fresh milk, use 1 quart of milk and add ½ cup of dry milk to create a thicker consistency. I always make plain yogurt, but if you would like to make sweetened yogurt, add ¼ cup of sugar or a couple of table-spoons of honey.

Heat milk very gently until it reaches 185°F. You can use a double boiler, or at the lowest possible setting over direct heat. This is an impor-tant step. You don't want to scald the milk or let it get too hot, so use a thermometer to check it.

Cool milk to about 110°F by placing it in a cool water bath. 110°F is slightly warm on the wrist, but it should not sting or tingle. Too hot and you may kill the live culture.

If you are using fresh yogurt, take it out of the refrigerator for a few minutes to warm up before adding to the milk. Stir it in to milk to blend. If you are using yogurt starter, follow package instructions.

Place milk in any kind of glass jar with a lid. Some people like to make enough to fill up a 1 quart jar, but I prefer to use four ½ pint jars.

Your yogurt mixture now needs to sit quietly in a warm place for several hours. Choose a location where the yogurt will not be moved or disturbed. Plan on about eight hours for yogurt to thicken.

You can incubate your yogurt in a number of ways. The key is to maintain a temperature of about 110–115°F at all times. This may take a little trial and error. A successful batch of yogurt will be slightly thickened and creamy. It will continue to thicken as it cools, so don't be alarmed if it is not quite as thick as you expect.

- Place an electric heating pad on the lowest setting and cover with a towel. Place yogurt mixture on top and cover the whole thing with a large towel. This is my preferred method because I find it to be very consistent.
- Place yogurt mixture in a pre-heated thermos and close tightly.
- Place jars of yogurt in a cooler filled with warm water.
- Place yogurt in an unheated gas oven with just the pilot light on. Electric ovens generally are hard to control under 200°F, so the environment may become too hot.

When your yogurt is ready, refrigerate it to finish thickening before using. Homemade yogurt should keep well in your refrigerator for a week or two.

Hot Chocolate Mix
 4 cups dry milk
 1 cup unsweetened cocoa
 2 cups sugar
 ½ teaspoon salt
 1 teaspoon instant coffee (optional)

Mix the ingredients and put them into a glass jar with a tight-fitting lid. Use ¼ cup per one cup of boiling water.

Chocolate Pudding Mix
 2½ cups dry milk
 5 cups sugar
 3 cups cornstarch
 1 teaspoon salt
 2½ cups cocoa powder

Mix all ingredients together until they are well blended. Store in a glass jar with a tight lid.

To make pudding, combine ⅔ cup of mix with 2 cups milk, one teaspoon vanilla, and one tablespoon butter. Cook over low heat, bringing gently to a boil. Cook and stir for one minute. Cool and serve.

Baking Soda

Baking soda is good for more than baking. It is great for deodorizing almost anything, works as an acid neutralizer, and can even stop an itch.

- Mix it in your bath water for a deodorizing cleanse.
- Make a paste with it for brushing your teeth and freshening your breath.
- Stir a little baking soda into water to make a soothing drink to counteract an upset stomach.
- Use a dash of baking soda under the arms as a replacement for deodorant.
- Apply a paste of baking soda and water to stings and bites to reduce itching.
- Add baking soda to laundry to eliminate smells and loosen stains.
- Sprinkle baking soda on a burned pot to loosen the char. Let sit a few minutes, and then scrub and rinse.
- A little baking soda instead of powder in the diaper can help neutralize ammonia.

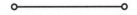

Sprouting Seeds

Sprouted seeds are very nutritious and are a wonderful way to produce fresh green vegetables from your dry pantry. To start, buy good quality sprouting seeds. These seeds are dormant when you get them, and can be kept that way for as much as five years if you give them the right conditions. Like most of the rest of your pantry, sprouting seeds need cool, dry, dark conditions.

Choose a sprouting vessel that will make it easy to rinse and drain your seeds. A simple canning jar with a mesh lid works well, or you can use more sophisticated sprouting trays. When you are ready to do some sprouting, take a quick look through your seeds for small stones or dirt and pick them out. Once they are clean, you are ready to soak them. Different seeds require different soaking times—a range between twenty minutes and several hours. Use a ratio of about 3:1; that is three times as much water as seed. Stir them up to make sure all the seeds have a chance to soak up some water. When they have finished soaking, drain all the water and discard it.

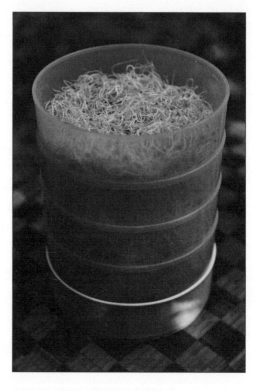

Place your sprouting container in an open room where it can receive fresh air. I just leave it on my kitchen counter near the sink so I won't forget to rinse it. Sprouts need air to perform their magic, so don't store them in a dark closet. Room light is fine and will help them to start greening when they are ready.

Thoroughly rinse your seeds with cool, fresh water two or three times a day and drain them after each rinsing, giving your container an extra shake or two to remove as much water as possible. Depending on conditions, sprouts are ready to eat in three to four days. If you are going to store your fresh sprouts in the refrigerator, make sure they are dry. Damp sprouts will not keep well.

Growing Wheat Grass

Wheat grass is highly nutritious and easy to grow on your kitchen windowsill. Just take some of your whole wheat berries—the same ones you have stored for grinding flour—and plant them in seed trays or a flower pot. Plant the berries in shallow ground, with just a thin layer of soil over them. Water well. You may harvest about an inch at a time. The grass will start to die off after a couple of weeks. Re-seed and start again.

Wheatgrass juice is highly prized for its nutritional, cleansing, and detoxification properties. To make pure wheatgrass juice, a special wheatgrass blender provides the best results.

A simple way to use wheatgrass that has always been popular with our kids is to simply throw a handful of chopped grass in the blender with some juice and ice cubes. This makes a frothy, refreshing, and very healthy summertime drink.

Using Dehydrated Vegetables

Although many convenience foods are nothing more than a combination of dried ingredients, dehydrated vegetables may be somewhat unfamiliar to the average home cook. I wasn't sure how I felt about dehydrated vegetables until I started using them regularly. I quickly discovered that they are not only highly nutritious, they are also really handy for making a quick soup or side dish. With dehydrated vegetables, there is no waste, no peeling or chopping, so soups, stews, and casseroles go together in a snap.

The texture of dehydrated vegetables is a little different than that of canned or frozen vegetables. If you are using the product alone, you may notice the difference. If you are adding it to a recipe with several other ingredients, you won't notice a thing.

Dehydrated vegetables can be reconstituted by soaking them in cool water or broth before cooking, or if you are making a recipe with plenty of liquid, like a soup or stew, they can be added directly into the pot along with your other ingredients. Dried greens and tomatoes do not need to be soaked ahead of time.

To sauté dehydrated vegetables, reconstitute them with a little less water than you might normally use. You want the vegetable to be soft, but not soggy, before adding them to the oil or butter.

Dehydrated Vegetable Equivalents
   1 whole onion = ¼ cup dried minced onions
   1 clove garlic = ¼ teaspoon dried garlic
   1 green pepper = ¼ cup green pepper flakes
   1 cup carrots = ½ cup dried carrots
   1 cup spinach = ½ cup dried spinach
   1 cup tomato = ½ cup dried tomatoes
   1 medium tomato = 1 tablespoon powdered tomato

Simple Vegetable Stew
   10 cups water
   1 teaspoon tomato powder
   1 teaspoon dried oregano
   1 teaspoon dried parsley
   ½ teaspoon garlic powder
   3 tablespoons beef bouillon granules
   ½ cup dehydrated carrots
   ½ cup dehydrated onions
   ½ cup dehydrated green bell peppers
   ½ cup dehydrated celery
   ½ cup potato dices
   ½ cup dehydrated peas
   ½ cup rice
   1 15-ounce can garbanzo beans, rinsed and drained

Combine all ingredients into a soup pot. Bring to a boil, reduce the heat, and simmer for thirty minutes. Add in rice and continue cooking until tender.

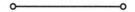

Textured Vegetable Protein

An excellent substitute for ground meats and something that makes a great source of protein in the dry pantry is textured vegetable protein (TVP). TVP is made from soy and is very shelf-stable. Plain TVP has been around for many years, but in recent times, many flavored versions have come on the market, including bacon, pepperoni, and sausage flavors.

To reconstitute TVP for use in recipes that call for ground meat, such as tacos, pour 3/4 of a cup of boiling water over 1 cup of TVP. Let stand for five to ten minutes, and then season and cook as you normally would. If you are adding it to a soup or stew, it can be added dry right into the pot.

TVP Sloppy Joes

    2 tablespoons vegetable oil
    1 medium onion, chopped
    1 medium green pepper, chopped
    2 teaspoons chili powder
    2 tablespoons tomato paste
    1/4 cup BBQ sauce
    2 tablespoons ketchup
    2 teaspoons mustard
    3/4 cup TVP
    3/4 cup boiling water
    Salt and pepper

Sauté the onion and green pepper in oil until vegetables are softened. Add all ingredients and simmer for twenty minutes.

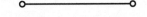

Food Substitutions

Inevitably there will come a time when you just don't have the ingredient you're looking for. Fortunately, there are many ways to make what you need using on-hand ingredients or substitutions.

Milk made from rice, for example, can make an acceptable milk substitute. It's good for any recipe calling for milk, and can be consumed by babies with upset tummies or folks who are lactose intolerant.

Rice Milk

Place 4 cups of water, 1 cup of cooked brown rice, and 1 teaspoon of vanilla in a blender and combine until very smooth. For clear milk, strain the resulting purée twice, first through a mesh strainer and then through a cheesecloth.

Common Substitutions

DON'T HAVE	USE INSTEAD
Baking:	
1 cup baking mix	1¾ cups all-purpose flour + 2½ tsp baking powder + ¾ tsp salt + ⅓ cup shortening
1 cup self-rising corn or white flour	1 cup flour + 1½ tsp baking powder + ½ tsp salt
1 tsp baking powder	¼ tsp baking soda, + ½ tsp cream of tartar, ¼ tsp baking soda, + ½ cup sour milk or plain yogurt
1 tbsp cornstarch	2 tbsp flour
1 oz square baking chocolate	3 tbsp cocoa powder + 1 tbsp butter
1 cup butter	¾ cup oil
1 egg	2 tbsp milk + ½ tsp baking powder
SUGAR	
1 cup corn syrup	1 cup sugar + ¼ cup water
1 cup brown sugar	1 cup sugar + 1-2 tbsp molasses
1 cup powdered sugar	1 cup sugar + 1 tsp cornstarch, ground in blender
1 cup sugar	¾ cup honey + 4 tbsp flour and ¼ tsp baking soda
Pancake syrup	½ cup brown sugar + 1½ cups water + 2½ tsp cornstarch. Cook until slightly thickened.

DAIRY	
1 cup buttermilk	1 cup milk + 1 tbsp lemon juice or vinegar, steeped for 5 minutes
1 cup heavy cream	1 cup evaporated milk
1 cup sour cream	¾ cup milk, soured with 1 tbsp lemon juice + 3 tbsp butter
1 cup sweetened condensed milk	1 cup nonfat dry milk + ½ cup boiling water +⅔ cup sugar + 3 tbsp melted butter (process in blender until smooth)
HERBS AND SPICES	
1 tbsp fresh herbs	½-1 tsp dried herbs
1 small onion	1 tbsp minced dried onion
1 clove garlic	⅛ tsp garlic powder or ¼ tsp dried minced garlic
1 tsp grated ginger root	¾ tsp ground ginger
1 tsp lemon juice	½ tsp vinegar
OTHER	
1 cup flavored gelatin	1 tbsp plain gelatin + 2 cups fruit juice
1 ketchup	1 cup tomato sauce + ½ cup sugar + 2 tbsp vinegar
1 cup tomato juice	½ cup tomato sauce + ½ cup water

Recipes from Your Pantry

Snacks

Roasted Wheat Berries
    1 tablespoon oil
    ½ cup wheat berries
    Salt

Heat oil in a cast iron skillet. Add wheat berries and toast, shaking the pan until all the berries are popped. The popping action is a little like popcorn, although don't expect much expansion. Remove from heat and immediately sprinkle with salt.

Toasted Cereal Mix
    ¼ cup butter
    1 tablespoon Worcestershire sauce
    1 teaspoon paprika
    1 teaspoon garlic salt
    4 cups unsweetened breakfast cereal
    2 cups pretzel sticks
    1 cup salted peanuts

Melt butter over low heat. Remove from heat and stir in sauce, paprika, and garlic salt.

Place cereal, pretzels, and peanuts in a large bowl. Pour melted butter over the dry ingredients and toss to coat. Bake at 275°F for about thirty minutes, stirring to toast cereal evenly.

Parmesan Corn

4 cups warm popped corn
1 tablespoon melted butter
½ cup grated Parmesan cheese
⅛ teaspoon cayenne pepper

Drizzle melted butter on warm popcorn. (You can spritz a little vegetable oil on the popped corn if you prefer.) Mix cayenne pepper with Parmesan cheese. Sprinkle mixture onto popcorn and toss until coated.

Kettle Corn

½ cup vegetable oil for popping
½ cup unpopped popcorn
4 tablespoons sugar
½ teaspoon salt

Heat oil in a medium saucepan. Add popcorn and watch until the kernels swell and begin to pop. Once one or two kernels have popped, sprinkle sugar on top. Quickly cover the saucepan and shake continuously until the corn stops popping. It may take a few moments for the corn to resume popping after the sugar is added. Remove corn and lay out on a cookie sheet to cool. Break large clusters apart, add salt, and toss to coat.

Hummus

1 15-ounce can garbanzo beans, rinsed and drained
1/4 cup lemon juice
1 tablespoon olive oil
2 cloves garlic

Process the beans and garlic in a food processor until they are puréed. Pour in the lemon juice and olive oil, continuing to purée until very smooth. Serve with crackers or vegetable sticks.

Energy Balls

½ cup peanut butter
¼ cup honey

½ teaspoon vanilla

1 cup old fashioned rolled oats

½ cup wheat germ

¼ cup dried cranberries

¼ cup chocolate chips

½ cup shredded coconut

Mix together peanut butter, honey, and vanilla. Stir in additional ingredients and form into a firm dough. Chill for about a half hour to make dough easy to work, then form smaller balls from it and roll them in shredded coconut if desired.

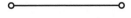

Breakfast

Baked Oatmeal

1½ cups quick-cooking oatmeal

½ cup brown sugar

½ cup milk

¼ cup melted butter

1 egg

1 teaspoon baking powder

½ teaspoon salt

1 teaspoon vanilla

Combine all ingredients and spread into a lightly oiled 9 x 13 inch baking dish. Bake for thirty minutes. Edges should be golden brown. Serve topped with cream, fruit, or maple syrup.

Almond Maple Granola

6 cups regular rolled oats

1 cup sliced almonds

½ cup raw sunflower seeds

1 cup unsweetened shredded or flaked coconut

¼ cup flax seeds

¼ cup sesame seeds

½ cup raw wheat germ

1 cup maple syrup
2 tablespoon vegetable oil
1 teaspoon vanilla extract

Mix oats, almonds, sunflower seeds, coconut, flax seeds, sesame seeds, and wheat germ in a large bowl. Combine maple syrup, water, oil, and vanilla, and pour over the dry ingredients. Toss until evenly coated. Spread the granola onto a cookie sheet and toast in the oven at 350°F for thirty to forty minutes, stirring occasionally to ensure even toasting. Remove from baking sheet and let cool before storing in an airtight container.

Muesli

2 cups oatmeal
1 cup milk
1 tablespoon honey
¼ cup slivered almonds
¼ cup dried unsweetened coconut flakes
¼ cup raisins
1 apple, peeled and grated
1 cup plain yogurt

Mix oatmeal, milk, and honey in a bowl and refrigerate overnight. In the morning, add almonds, coconut, raisins, and apples. Stir in yogurt to coat.

Blueberry Quinoa Porridge

½ cup uncooked quinoa
1 cup water
½ teaspoon cinnamon
Pinch of salt
½ cup milk
½ cup blueberries
1 tablespoon brown sugar

Place quinoa, water, cinnamon, and salt in a small pot and bring to a boil. Reduce heat, cover and simmer for about fifteen minutes. Uncover, add milk, and continue to simmer for another ten minutes or so. Stir in blueberries and brown sugar. Cover and let sit for ten minutes before serving. Garnish with sliced almonds or walnuts.

Oatmeal Pancakes

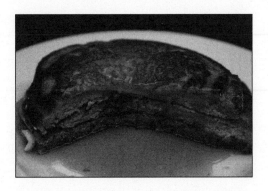

    1 cup milk
    1¼ cups old-fashioned
    oatmeal
    2 eggs
    1 tablespoon vegetable oil
    ½ cup whole wheat flour
    2 tablespoons brown sugar
    1 teaspoon baking powder
    ¼ teaspoon salt

Place oatmeal in a bowl and cover with milk. Stir and allow oats to soak in milk for about five minutes. Stir in eggs and oil and then mix in flour, sugar, baking powder, and salt. Cook pancakes on heated, oiled griddle. Serve with fresh applesauce or sliced bananas.

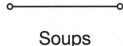

Soups

Easy Southwestern Soup

    1 15-oz can whole kernel corn, drained
    4 cups chicken broth
    1 15-oz can black beans
    1 10-oz can diced tomatoes
    1 4-oz can diced green chilies

Pour all ingredients into a large pot and simmer for thirty minutes, or until heated through.

Fast Minestrone

    6 cups chicken broth
    1 cup V8 juice
    1 cup canned tomatoes, diced
    2 tablespoons onion flakes
    ¼ teaspoon garlic powder
    1 teaspoon dried oregano
    ½ teaspoon dried thyme

1 cup cooked elbow noodles, rice, or orzo
1 15-oz can cannellini beans, drained and rinsed
1 15-oz can sliced carrots, drained
1 15-oz can cut green beans, drained
1 4-oz can sliced mushrooms, drained Parmesan cheese, grated

Stir broth, vegetable juice, and tomatoes together. Add all the seasonings. Bring to a boil, then reduce to a simmer. Cook for thirty minutes. Stir in your choice of cooked starch, along with beans, carrots, green beans, and mushrooms. Heat until warmed through, adding more chicken stock if needed. Serve sprinkled with grated Parmesan.

Carrot and Apple Soup
½ stick butter
1 tablespoon fresh ginger, grated
2 tablespoons soy sauce
2 apples, sliced
2 cups carrots, peeled and sliced
1 tablespoon lemon juice
3 cups vegetable stock
2 cups yogurt
Salt and pepper

Sauté ginger in melted butter with soy sauce, stirring until smooth and bubbly. Add apples, carrots, and lemon juice, and toss in butter to coat all ingredients. Add 2 cups of vegetable stock and cook until carrots are very tender, about thirty minutes. Remove from heat and cool slightly, then purée carrot mixture in blender, adding 1 more cup of stock. Return purée to pot and fold in yogurt. Heat very gently, season with salt and pepper.

Blender Soup
4 cups milk
2 cups re-hydrated vegetables
4 tablespoons flour
4 tablespoons oil
Salt, pepper, seasonings

Blend all ingredients together. Heat slightly or serve at room temperature with a dollop of sour cream and a garnish of chopped chives. This soup is really tasty and endlessly versatile. Try a combination of potato, onion, and spinach with thyme, or corn and red peppers with a dash of cumin, or plain green peas with mint leaves. Season as desired.

Bread Soup

    4 thick slices French bread
    3 cloves garlic, peeled and sliced
    1 medium onion, finely chopped
    ¼ cup olive oil
    12 fresh basil leaves, chopped
    2 pounds Roma tomatoes, peeled and diced
    4 cups chicken stock
    1 teaspoon salt
    ¼ teaspoon black pepper
    Parmesan cheese, grated

Place bread on grill or in oven. Don't toast it, just dry it out. Break bread into large pieces and set aside. Sauté the garlic and onion in olive oil until soft; be careful not to brown them.

Stir basil and tomatoes into a pot with the garlic and onion and simmer for fifteen to twenty minutes. Add chicken stock, bread, salt, and pepper, and continue to simmer for another fifteen to twenty minutes. Stir occasionally to break down the bread and incorporate it into the broth. Sprinkle with freshly grated Parmesan cheese and serve.

TVP Chili

    1 cup textured vegetable protein
    1 cup beef stock
    2 tablespoons vegetable oil
    1 medium onion, chopped
    2 cloves garlic, minced
    1 8-ounce can tomato sauce
    1 15-ounce can diced tomatoes
    1½ cups water
    2 tablespoons chili powder

1 teaspoon cumin

1 teaspoon Mexican oregano

1 15-ounce can black beans, rinsed and drained

Salt and pepper

Bring beef stock to a boil and pour it over the TVP. Set aside to soak. Place oil in a pan and sauté onion and garlic until softened. Add in reconstituted TVP, tomato sauce, tomatoes, water, spices, and black beans. Simmer for thirty minutes, uncovered.

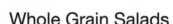

Whole Grain Salads

Rice and Bean Sprout Salad

1½ cups cooked brown rice

½ cup fresh parsley, chopped

1 cup canned pineapple, drained and chopped

4 green onions, whites and greens chopped

½ cup radishes, thinly sliced

½ cup pecans, roughly chopped

1 cup fresh bean sprouts

Dressing

4 tablespoons olive oil

1 tablespoon lemon juice

1 tablespoon apple cider vinegar

1 tablespoon dry mustard

1 tablespoon powdered ginger

1 tablespoon honey

Salt and pepper

Combine the dressing ingredients in a jar and shake until thoroughly blended. Place rice, parsley, pineapple, green onions, radishes, pecans, and sprouts into a bowl. Pour dressing over the mix and toss until well-coated.

Kitchen Sink Salad

4 cups cooked whole wheat spirals

1 15-ounce can canned red kidney beans, drained and rinsed

4 green onions, white and greens sliced

2 celery stalks, chopped

1 small red bell pepper, diced

1 medium cucumber, peeled and diced

1 carrot, peeled and diced

1 cup baby spinach leaves, chopped

½ cup sliced ripe olives

3 marinated artichoke hearts, chopped

Cherry tomatoes, halved

Dressing

1 cup sour cream

2 tablespoons cider vinegar

1 teaspoon sugar

1 teaspoon salt

½ teaspoon celery seed

1 teaspoon dried basil

Combine pasta, kidney beans, and the rest of the salad ingredients in a bowl. Choose whatever you have available—at my house, this recipe is rarely the same twice. Throw in your own favorite chopped vegetables and add protein in the form of cheese, bacon, ham, or hard boiled eggs, if you like.

Make dressing by whisking together sour cream, vinegar, sugar, and seasonings; shake to combine. Pour dressing over pasta and toss.

Quinoa Salad

¾ cup dry quinoa, cooked

1½ cups water

1 bunch green onions, whites and greens sliced

1 cup diced red bell pepper

1 medium cucumber, peeled and diced

1 cup canned black beans, drained and rinsed

1 cup corn

3 tablespoons cider vinegar

2 tablespoons olive oil

1 tablespoon sugar

½ teaspoon salt

¼ teaspoon pepper

Cook quinoa in lightly salted water for about fifteen minutes. Set aside to cool.

In a large bowl, combine cooked quinoa, green onions, bell pepper, cucumber black beans, and corn. Make dressing by whisking together vinegar, oil, sugar, salt, and black pepper; shake to combine. Pour dressing over quinoa salad and toss.

Wild Rice Salad with Cranberries and Walnuts

1 cup wild rice, rinsed

2 cups chicken stock

2 cups water

4 green onions, whites and greens sliced

1 cup frozen peas, thawed

1 cup dried cranberries

½ cup walnut pieces

1 large apple, cored and chopped

1 tablespoon lemon juice

Dressing

½ cup olive oil

½ cup cider vinegar

2 teaspoons honey

Salt and pepper to taste

Place wild rice, chicken stock, and water in a pot. Bring to a boil and then reduce to simmer. Cook rice, covered, for about forty-five minutes. Drain and transfer to a bowl to cool. In a small bowl, toss chopped apple with lemon juice to prevent browning.

When rice is cool, add onions, peas, cranberries, walnuts, and chopped apples. Make dressing by whisking together oil, vinegar, honey, salt, and pepper. Pour dressing over wild rice, tossing to coat thoroughly. Refrigerate several hours before serving.

Tabouli

1 cup bulgur

1½ cups boiling water

1 bunch green onions, greens and whites chopped

2 cups fresh parsley, chopped
½ cup fresh mint, chopped
½ cup olive oil
½ cup lemon juice
Salt and pepper to taste
1 cucumber, peeled and diced
2 medium tomatoes, diced

Place clean bulgur in a bowl and pour boiling water over it. Set aside for about thirty minutes.

While bulgur is soaking, chop vegetables and make dressing by whisking oil, lemon juice, salt, and pepper together.

Drain bulgur, pressing it to the side of the bowl with a wooden spoon to remove excess water. Stir in onions, parsley, and mint. Pour in dressing and toss thoroughly to coat grain. Add diced cucumber and tomatoes. Let stand at room temperature for a couple of hours before serving.

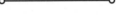

Main Dishes

Grainy Grain Casserole
2 tablespoons olive oil
1 small onion, chopped
1 small red bell pepper, chopped
2 medium carrots, cut into thin slices
1 cup mushrooms, sliced
1 clove garlic, finely chopped
1 15-oz can diced tomatoes with juice
1 cup fresh or frozen corn
¼ cup fresh spinach, chopped
2 cups cooked black beans, drained and rinsed
½ cup uncooked pearl barley
¼ cup uncooked bulgur wheat
½ cup chicken stock
1 teaspoon dried oregano

¼ teaspoon salt

¼ teaspoon pepper

Place oil in a heavy-bottomed saucepan. Add onions and pepper, and sauté until softened. Add carrots, mushrooms, and garlic. Stir in tomatoes, corn, spinach, black beans, barley, bulgur, and stock. Season with oregano, salt, and pepper. Transfer to a lightly oiled casserole dish, cover, and bake at 350°F for one hour.

Almond Stir Fry

3 tablespoons vegetable oil

2 large onions, thinly sliced

2 cloves garlic, minced

3 carrots, peeled and thinly sliced

3 stalks celery, thinly sliced

1 cup mushrooms, sliced

2 cups mung bean sprouts

1 cup whole natural almonds

1 cup stir-fry sauce

Stir Fry Sauce

½ cup cornstarch

¼ cup brown sugar

2 teaspoons dried ginger

½ dried garlic

½ teaspoon cayenne

½ cup soy sauce

¼ cup cider vinegar

2 cups chicken or vegetable stock

½ cup water

To make stir fry sauce: Combine cornstarch, brown sugar, ginger, garlic, and cayenne. Add soy sauce and vinegar, whisking until blended. Add stock and water, stirring until smooth.

Place oil in wok and heat. Add onions, garlic, carrots, and celery, stirring to coat with oil. When carrots start to soften, add mushrooms, bean sprouts, and almonds. Cook and stir until the vegetables are al dente. Add 1 cup of the stir fry sauce and continue cooking until sauce has coated all ingredients. Save leftover sauce in the refrigerator for up to two weeks.

Serve over cooked rice or millet.

Oat Flakes and Sunflower Casserole
2 tablespoons vegetable oil
2 cups freshly ground oat flakes
¼ teaspoon salt
2½ cups water
2 tablespoons vegetable oil
1 large onion, chopped
1 stalk celery, chopped
1 green bell pepper, chopped
2 cloves garlic, minced
2 tablespoons fresh parsley, chopped
½ cup raw sunflower seeds
2 tablespoons soy sauce
1 teaspoon cumin

Sauté oat flakes in oil for five minutes and then add water and salt. Cover and simmer on low heat for twenty minutes or until softened.

While oats are cooking, sauté vegetables and sunflower seeds in oil. Combine the sautéed vegetables and seeds with the cooked oat flakes. Stir in soy sauce and cumin.

Transfer everything to a lightly oiled two-quart casserole dish. Bake for thirty minutes at 350°F. Serve topped with béchamel sauce.

Béchamel Sauce
¼ cup oil
1 cup whole wheat flour
4 cups water
¼ cup soy sauce

Heat oil in a saucepan. Gently stir in flour, stirring to toast until it is golden brown and smells a little nutty. Set aside to cool.

When flour is cool, whisk in water and salt. Bring to a boil, and then reduce heat and simmer until thickened. Stir in soy sauce and continue to cook for another five minutes. Store leftover sauce in the refrigerator.

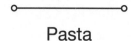

Pasta

Whole Wheat Spaghetti with Edamame and Spinach
  2 tablespoons olive oil
  ¼ cup pine nuts
  2 cloves garlic, sliced
  4 cups cooked spaghetti, drained and tossed with a splash of olive oil
  2 cups shelled edamame, cooked and drained
  4 cups spinach, chopped
  ½ cup grated Parmesan cheese

Place oil in a large sauté pan and add pine nuts, cooking gently to toast. Add garlic, being careful not to let it brown. Toss in cooked spaghetti, edamame, and spinach leaves, adding another splash of olive oil if needed. Cook until spinach is limp and incorporated into pasta. Toss Parmesan into pasta and serve.

Spinach Fettuccine with Tuna Sauce
  ½ cup olive oil
  1 large onion, chopped
  2 cloves garlic, minced
  1 large red bell pepper, chopped
  1 28-oz can Italian Roma tomatoes, drained
  Salt and pepper to taste
  1 12-oz can tuna packed in oil, drained
  1 pound spinach fettuccine, cooked, drained, and tossed with olive oil

Place oil in a heavy-bottomed pan and sauté onions, garlic, and bell peppers until softened. Add tomatoes and season with salt and pepper. Simmer for fifteen minutes, using the back of a wooden spoon to crush tomatoes slightly. Stir in tuna and continue to cook just to heat tuna through.

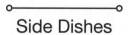

Side Dishes

Brown Rice Fritters
  2 cups cooked brown rice
  ½ cup grated Parmesan

1 egg
½ teaspoon salt
A couple of grinds of black pepper
½ cup flour
¼ cup vegetable oil

Combine rice, cheese, egg, salt, and pepper. Form into patties and place in refrigerator to chill. When ready to cook, dredge each patty in flour and cook in pre-heated oil, turning once to brown, three to four minutes per side.

Spanish Rice

2 tablespoons butter
1 medium onion, chopped
1 red bell pepper, seeded and diced
1 clove garlic, minced
1 cup white rice
2 cups chicken stock
1 large tomato, seeded and chopped
1 jalapeno, seeded and diced
2 teaspoons chili powder
1 teaspoon ground cumin

Place butter in a heavy-bottomed saucepan. Sauté onions, bell pepper, and garlic, cooking until softened. Add the rice, stirring until lightly golden. Add stock, tomato, jalapeno, chili powder, and cumin. Cover and simmer for five minutes.

Pour rice mixture into a buttered one-quart casserole. Bake at 375°F or until the stock is fully absorbed, about forty minutes.

Scalloped Green Beans

2 15-oz cans green beans, drained
1 10-oz can cream of mushroom soup
½ cup milk
½ cup dried bread crumbs
1 tablespoon butter

Combine beans, soup, and milk together and place in a buttered casserole dish. Melt butter and mix into bread crumbs. Top beans with bread crumbs. Bake at 350°F for twenty minutes or until beans are bubbly and crust is browned.

Stir-fried Ramen Noodles

1 3-oz package ramen soup noodles with flavor packet
2 tablespoons olive oil
½ cup chopped onion
½ cup chopped celery
1 clove garlic, minced
1 cup frozen peas, thawed

Cook the ramen noodles in boiling water, then drain and set aside. Place oil in a wok and add onions, celery, and garlic. Sauté until softened. Stir in the flavor packet and add the cooked noodles and peas. Toss until coated and serve topped with Parmesan cheese.

Savory Bread Pudding

4 large eggs
2 cups milk
½ teaspoon Tabasco sauce
½ teaspoon salt
½ teaspoon black pepper
3½ cups stale bread, cubed
1 tablespoon olive oil
1 medium onion, chopped
1 green bell pepper, chopped
1 clove garlic, minced
2 cups mushrooms, chopped
2 cups fresh spinach, chopped

In a bowl, whisk together milk, eggs, Tabasco sauce, salt, and pepper. Stir the bread cubes into the egg mixture and set aside. Place oil in a large sauté pan. Add onions and bell pepper and stir until softened. Add mushrooms and garlic, stirring until moisture from mushrooms has evaporated. Stir in spinach, and cook until it wilts. Add the cooked vegetables to the bread and egg mixture, stirring until thoroughly blended. Move the mixture into a greased casserole dish. Cover the baking dish with foil and bake until the pudding is set in the center, about an hour. Uncover the dish and bake for an additional 10 minutes.

Rice and Peas

 1 small onion, chopped
 1 small red bell pepper, chopped
 2 tablespoons olive oil
 4 cups cooked white rice
 1 cup frozen peas, thawed
 ½ cup slivered almonds
 1 tablespoon chopped parsley
 2 green onions, sliced
 Salt and pepper to taste

In a large, heavy saucepan, cook the onions and bell peppers in the olive oil over medium heat for three to four minutes, or until slightly soft. Add the rice, peas, and almonds and stir to mix. Remove from the heat and season with salt and black pepper. Add the parsley and green onions. Serve warm.

Fried Corn

 2 tablespoons butter or bacon drippings
 4 cups frozen corn, thawed
 1 red bell pepper, diced
 1 small onion, diced
 1 teaspoon white flour
 ½ cup milk
 2 tablespoons fresh chopped parsley
 Salt and pepper to taste

Heat bacon drippings in a large skillet until just sizzling. Add corn, bell pepper, and onions, and sauté until corn begins to brown. Sprinkle flour over corn and stir to incorporate. Stir in cream. Salt and pepper to taste.

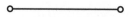

Breads

Tex-Mex Cornbread

1½ cups cornmeal
1 cup milk
¾ teaspoon salt
½ cup melted butter
½ teaspoon baking soda
1 14-oz can cream-style corn
6 green onions, whites and greens diced
1 4-oz can diced green chilies

Mix together cornmeal, milk, salt, butter, soda, and canned corn. Pour half the batter into a lightly oiled round 10-inch pan. Layer the onions and green chilies over the batter. Pour the rest of the batter on top. Bake at 350°F for thirty-five to forty minutes.

Soda Bread

3½ cups flour
1 teaspoon sugar
1 teaspoon salt
1 teaspoon baking soda
1 cup buttermilk

Preheat the Dutch oven to 350°F. Mix flour, sugar, salt, and baking soda together in a bowl to thoroughly combine. Add buttermilk a little at a time and continue to stir until a soft dough forms. Transfer to a lightly floured board and knead very lightly. Form the dough into a round dome. With a sharp knife, cut a cross on the top of the circle and about halfway down the sides. Lift gently and place into the Dutch oven. Cover and bake for thirty-five minutes. To test if it's done, pick up the loaf and tap the bottom. It should sound a little hollow. For a softer crust, wrap in a towel when the bread is cooling.

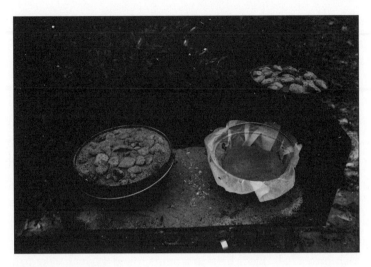

Zucchini Crown Rolls

2 cups zucchini, gratcd

Salt

5 cups flour

1 package yeast

¼ cup freshly grated Parmesan cheese

1 teaspoon salt

1 teaspoon black pepper

2 tablespoons olive oil

About 2 cups lukewarm water

Milk and sesame seeds for glaze

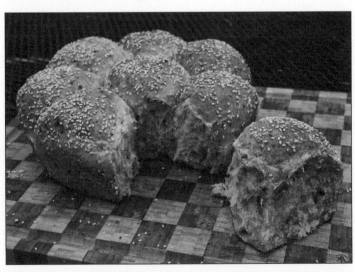

Grate the zucchini and sprinkle lightly with salt. Place in a colander to drain for about thirty minutes. Squeeze thoroughly and pat dry to remove excess moisture.

Mix together the flour, yeast, Parmesan, salt, and black pepper. Mix in the oil and zucchini. Stir in one cup water, and then add remaining water a little at a time, stirring until your dough is firm. Turn dough out of bowl and knead lightly, dusting with flour as needed. Place ball of dough in an oiled mixing bowl, turning it once to oil the top of dough. Cover with a towel and set in a sunny place to rise. Dough should double in size. Time for rising will vary. On a warm, sunny day, less than an hour should do it.

Punch down dough and knead it lightly. Cut it into eight equal pieces, rolling each into a ball. Place balls in a lightly oiled 12-inch cake pan. Brush the tops with milk and sprinkle with sesame seeds. Cover with towel and let rise for about thirty minutes. Bake at 350°F for thirty-five to forty minutes.

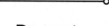

Desserts

Bread Pudding
> 8 cups day-old French bread, cut into 2-inch (5 cm) chunks
> ¾ cup raisins, soaked for 10 minutes in rum
> 1 cup chopped pecans
> 5 eggs
> ¾ cup sugar
> 2½ cups milk
> 2½ cups heavy cream
> 1 tablespoon vanilla
> ¾ teaspoon nutmeg
> ¼ teaspoon salt

Lightly butter a 12-inch baking dish. Toss bread, raisins, and nuts together and place in the Dutch oven. Beat eggs and sugar together. Blend in milk and cream and add vanilla, nutmeg, and salt. Pour over bread. Bake at 350°F for forty-five minutes or until the edges are golden and the center still shakes a little. Remove from oven and serve with whipped cream.

Ozark Pudding

1½ cups sugar

¼ cup all-purpose flour

2½ teaspoons baking powder

¼ teaspoon salt

2 eggs

1 teaspoon vanilla

1 medium apple, peeled and chopped

1 cup pecans, chopped

Beat sugar, flour, baking powder, salt, eggs, and vanilla together until smooth. Stir in apple and pecans. Pour batter into a lightly buttered 10-inch baking dish. Bake until top is browned, about forty minutes. Take the cake out of the oven immediately after cooking. Let cool a bit, but serve warm, preferably with whipped cream.

Autumn Cobbler

3 cups peeled, sliced apples

1 cup blackberries

½ cup brown sugar

½ cup flour

½ cup old-fashioned oats

1 teaspoon cinnamon

½ cup butter

Place sliced apples and blackberries in a lightly oiled 9-inch pan. Mix the rest of the ingredients into a soft crumble and sprinkle evenly over fruit. Bake at 350°F for about thirty minutes, or until the fruit is bubbly and the topping is golden brown.

Stovetop Rice Pudding

1½ cups leftover cooked white rice

2 cups milk, divided

⅓ cup sugar

¼ teaspoon cinnamon

¼ teaspoon salt

1 egg, beaten

½ cup dried cranberries

¼ cup pistachios
1 tablespoon butter
½ teaspoon vanilla

Place cooked rice in a saucepan and add 1 cup of milk, sugar, cinnamon, and salt. Cook on low heat for fifteen to twenty minutes, stirring until thick and creamy. Add the other cup of milk and beaten egg, stirring and cooking until egg is thoroughly incorporated, about two to three minutes. Stir in dried cranberries, pistachios, butter, and vanilla.

9

Growing, Gathering, and Preserving Your Own Food

There is an old saying that goes "If you give a man a fish, he will be able to feed himself for a day. But if you teach a man to fish, he can eat for the rest of his life." The same could be said for growing and gathering your own food. Providing for yourself through gardening, husbanding your own animals, or even learning to hunt provides a sense of confidence and self-sufficiency. Some of these skills may be impractical in the suburban setting, but even a small patio herb garden and a few tomato plants connect you to the source of your food in a practical way.

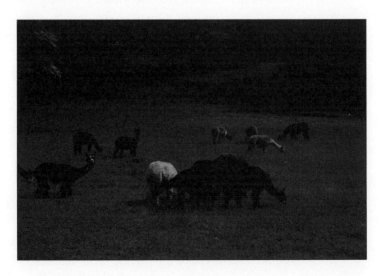

○———————○

Grow a Garden, Even in Small Spaces

If you already live in the country, chances are you already do some form of gardening. But if you live in the city, or even in the suburbs, you may not feel that you have the space to produce enough fruit and vegetables to be worth your while. The reality is, though, that even a small well-designed garden can produce enough to supplement your family's diet.

You can build a raised bed garden in as little as four square feet. "Square foot gardening," a high-yield, low space gardening method popularized by Mel Bartholomew in his book *Square Foot Gardening*, allows you to plant a different crop in each square foot of the garden. Four square feet gives you sixteen different options and will allow you to grow as much as you might produce in a garden over four times as big. What you put in each square depends on the spacing requirements of the plants you choose. You may put in one tomato, or use a square foot to plant nine green bean seeds. If you have more space, you can add additional boxes.

Choose a space for your garden that gets at least six to eight hours of sunshine. The quality of your soil isn't important. Your box will contain your own blend of soil.

- To create your garden, lay it out in squares that are no larger than four feet. If you are going to have more than one square, make room between them for walking. You will not be stepping into your squares once they are built.
- Construct boxes of 1 x 6 inch or 2 x 6 inch boards, connected at each corner with deck screws or corner brackets. Try to set the frames as level as possible, using soil to build up low areas. If you are positioning your boxes over grass or a weedy area, cover the ground with landscape paper or plastic to deter weeds.
- Make a rich, light blend of soil to fill your container. Make sure to add vermiculite to help hold the moisture. This is especially important in a shallow raised bed garden that will dry out faster than a conventional one.
- Choose and plant your vegetables. To understand how many seeds or plants to use per square, check the spacing recommendations on

the package. Seeds that call for 6-inch spacing can be planted four per square, 4-inch spacing can have nine per square. Plant one or two seeds in each spot, covering lightly with soil.

- Water every day when you first get started. After that, you may need to water daily only when it is very hot. Water early or late, rather than in the middle of the day when the sun can evaporate the water quickly.

- Harvest your crops as they come in. If a square gets emptied, replant it with another crop. If frost threatens, it is easy to construct posts to support the addition of a plastic cover over the box. This will turn it into a little hothouse that will help to extend your growing season.

○———————○

Herbs

Herbs add flavor and interest to your cooking and can also add to your home health care supply. Herbs have been used since the earliest times to counteract colds, heal injuries, and boost the immune system. We have long kept a potted aloe plant in our kitchen for burns. Calendula water makes a great antiseptic wash for minor cuts.

Herbs are classified as perennial, biennial, or annual, with perennials growing back throughout the year, biennials turning up every other year, and annuals being replaced yearly. Herbs are generally considered hardy or tender, so your climate and conditions may also dictate the management of your herb garden. Our garden includes a variety of perennial herbs, including mint and oregano, chives, rosemary, chamomile, lavender, sage, thyme, and tarragon. Echinacea and horseradish, which are grown for their roots, are given their own special area. Dill, cilantro, basil, garlic, and parsley are replenished yearly or as needed. We also grow salad greens such as savory, borage, sorrel, and lamb's quarters.

The best way to establish your herb garden is with seedlings from a local nursery. Choose an area with lots of sunlight where perennials will be allowed to flourish. (The exception is mint, which actually likes a shadier location.) If you have an herb that you use daily, the way we use chives, you can place a potted one near your kitchen door. You can also mix some perennials into your foundation plantings; we have rosemary growing as a hedge alongside our house. Most herbs just want reasonably good soil. Over-fertilizing them can make them rangy and unattractive.

Harvest your herbs often, before they flower. You can extend the life of your herbs by harvesting a little at a time, removing flowers as they form.

Air-drying Herbs

Fresh herbs are too delicate for direct sunlight, but they can easily be air-dried. Harvest and wash your herbs with stems. Lay out to dry on a towel, then gather into a bunch and tie the stems together. Hang upside down in a warm, dry place with good air circulation. Drying takes five or more days, depending on humidity and temperature conditions. Store dried herbs in airtight containers.

Cooking with Herbs

Fresh herbs can add flavor to salads and fresh sauces, and they make a beautiful garnish. When cooking with fresh herbs, a rule of thumb is that you need about three times as much fresh herbs as you would dried herbs. That means if a recipe calls for a teaspoon of a dried herbs, you would want three teaspoons (equally one tablespoon) instead. Chives, parsley, and rosemary are really best used fresh.

If you are cooking something that will simmer for thirty minutes or more, dried herbs will do just as well as fresh, particularly if they are your own dried herbs from that season. Dried herbs also work best for herb rubs.

Making Herbal Vinegar and Oil

Herb vinegars and herb-infused oils are a great base for vinaigrettes, mustards, marinades, and other sauces.

We usually keep at least a couple of different herb vinegars on hand. I like to make a mixed herb vinegar of sage, rosemary, and thyme as well as a mint vinegar. Garlic vinegar is also delicious, particularly combined with dried hot red chile peppers. To make herb vinegar, combine about a cup of fresh chopped herbs with two cups of vinegar. If you are making a fruit vinegar, try equal parts fruit and vinegar. Wine vinegars or apple cider vinegars are the most flavorful choices. Place your herbs in a clean bottle and cover with vinegar. Let it sit for at least a full day, although steeping it longer will enhance the flavor. Replace the vinegar as you use it so that the herbs are always covered. If you are adding garlic or scallions, clean and peel them before placing in the bottle. Garlic tends to float to the surface, so placing the cloves on a skewer is a good way to keep them where you want them. If you want to add chilies, stem and seed them before placing in the bottle.

To make herb-infused oil, the same practice applies. Place clean herbs, lightly bruised, into a bottle and cover with oil. Any good salad oil will work, but milder oils such as sunflower or light extra-virgin olive oil will let the flavor of the herbs shine through. Seal the bottle and place out of sunlight for a week or two to let the flavors emerge. I usually remove the herbs and strain the oil when it has reached the flavor I want. Garlic oil is usually strong enough after a few days; remove the cloves when it reaches its maturity. Oils are more fragile than you may believe, so I store all my oils in the refrigerator.

Herbal Soap

I love handmade soap. I buy interesting ones wherever I find them and love to make my own creations. My simple recipe is actually made with bars of soap, so the point of making it is mostly aesthetic—I get something fancier, more fragrant, and more customized at a lower cost. If you like the idea of making soap from more basic ingredients or are looking for a recipe that is strictly vegetarian, you can start with lye and oils to make your soaps.

This handmade soap recipe is very easy. All you need are some dried herbs, a plain soap bar (glycerin soap, Ivory soap, or any unscented soap will work), and a mold. To make herbal soap, place ¼ cup of boiling water with about a tablespoon of dried, crumbled herbs into a double boiler. Remove from heat and let steep for at least fifteen minutes. Return the water to the heat and add the bar of soap, crumbled or shredded into little pieces. Stir gently until the soap is melted and the herbs are evenly disbursed. Remove the liquid soap from the heat and pour it into lightly oiled molds. Let the soap cool until hardened and then remove it from the molds.

To make an exfoliating soap, add one tablespoon of ground oatmeal to melted soap before placing in the molds. For a scented soap, add a few drops of your favorite essential oil.

Herbal Cough Syrup

This is a simple cough syrup that can help to ease the tickle in your throat from a cold or hay fever. A honey-based syrup is much safer and just as effective as over-the-counter cough medicines, especially for children.

To make your own cough syrup, boil four cups of water along with about two ounces of a comforting herb. Fennel seed, Echinacea, thyme, anise, and wild cherry bark are common choices. Boil until water is reduced to two cups. Strain and add 3 tablespoons of honey. Cool the syrup and store it in a glass bottle.

If you prefer, make a soothing tea of the syrup by adding two tablespoons syrup to a cup of hot water.

Preserving Your Food

If you grow your own vegetables and fruit, or even if you are just a frequent visitor to the farmer's market, you may want to learn to preserve your own produce. Preserving it yourself allows you to customize salt and sweetening preferences to your family's needs and lets you put up favorite jam and pickle recipes. A shelf of home-canned foods is a very rewarding sight, and there is nothing like reaching for your own garden tomatoes on a cold winter's night.

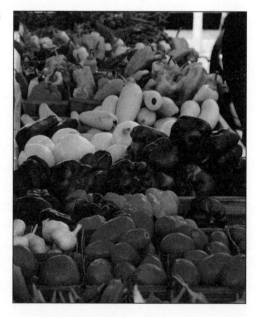

Water Bath Canning

Canning highly acidic produce, such as tomatoes and fruit, requires nothing more than a large water bath canner, along with canning jars with jar lids and screw bands. To can jams, jellies, pickles, fruit, and tomato products, follow these steps:

- Wash jars in hot, soapy water and set them aside to drain. It is okay to reuse any jar that fits your canning lid and screw top; just check the rim for smoothness and don't use any that are chipped or cracked. Fill the water bath canner with water and set it on the stove to simmer. Place jars on the rack and lower them into the hot water. The water does not have to boil.

- Place the new jar lids in a small saucepan. (Some say that jar lids can be reused, but I think it's safer to use new ones.) Add water and simmer on the stove. Screw bands should be clean, but do not have to be sterilized.

- Prepare your ingredients and make your recipe, if one is called for.

- When you are ready to fill the jars, work with one at a time. Take a hot jar from the pot and pour any excess water back into the pot. Using a jar funnel, fill the jar to within one-fourth to one-half inches of headspace.

- Using a chopstick or other non-metallic utensil, stir the ingredients of the jar so that everything settles and any air bubbles are released. If you need to add more ingredients or liquid to raise the level after settling your ingredients, do so now.

- Using a clean cloth, wipe down the rim of the jar so there is nothing blocking the seal. Center a hot jar lid on the top of the jar and tighten a screw band by hand. Place the jar back in the hot water. Repeat until all the jars are filled.

- When the jars are all filled and in the canner, add hot water until the level is about one inch over the top of the jars. Cover, turn up heat, and bring to a full rolling boil. When the water is boiling, begin counting the processing time. The water should continue to boil during the entire processing period.

- When the processing time is over, turn off the heat and remove the canner lid. Let jars sit inside for about five minutes, then place them on a towel-covered counter and cool.

- Wait several hours before checking to see whether your jars have sealed properly. To do this, remove the screw band and press down on the center of the lid. It should be slightly concave and not move when touched. The edge should hold tightly when pressure is applied. If a jar does not seal, just place it in the refrigerator and use within a few days.
- Store sealed and labeled jars in a cool, dark place. Home canned goods are best used within one year.
- To can low-acid vegetables or meats, a similar procedure is followed, but jars are processed in a pressure cooker to expose them to higher heat that can kill harmful bacterial spores. To can low-acid foods, read the pressure cooker manufacturer's directions and follow recipe instructions for processing times.

Pickling

Pickling has been used for centuries to preserve food. A high-acid environment is required to keep food from spoiling, so pickling generally involves salt, vinegar, or both. To make the preserving process even more foolproof, can the food using a water bath canner to remove the oxygen and create an airtight seal.

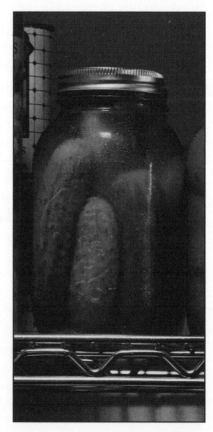

A wide array of foods can be preserved by pickling, from fish to eggs and fruits and vegetables. The basic process is the same for any food item. Heat your brine mixture of vinegar and salt, and then pour it over your food and seal. The freshly brined food must be set aside for several days or weeks in order to make sure the vinegar and salt have been fully incorporated into the food.

Although the first thing you associate with pickles is the cucumber, I find that it is actually the pickled food I like least. Dilly beans, sweet pickled cauliflower, and pickled asparagus spears are some of my family's favorites.

Fresh-Pack Pickles

It is important that the brine mixture recipe is suited to the type of vegetable or food item you are pickling, so follow your recipe carefully. For example, a 1:1 ratio of vinegar to water is common for cucumbers, but for pickled peppers, you will find that the recipe calls for a higher ratio of vinegar. This type of fresh-pack pickle generally calls for salt to aid in the preservation process, but salt is not absolutely necessary for all fresh pickles, so if you prefer a low-salt version, there are recipes available. Any type of vinegar can be used, but its acidity must be 5 percent to make sure that it will safely preserve your food. Recipes may call for sugar as well as herbs, spices, or garlic.

Pickling salt is required for making pickles. Pickling salt does not contain iodine or the anti-caking ingredients that are in common table salt. Table salt will produce a well-preserved pickle, but it may be cloudy and darker than one made with the correct salt. There are two secrets to good dill pickles. The first is to pickle within twenty-four hours of picking. The fresher the cucumber, the crisper the pickle. The second secret is soaking. Always soak your cucumbers in ice water to get a good crisp pickle.

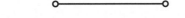

Old-Fashioned Dill Pickles

8 pounds pickling cucumbers
4 cups white vinegar
12 cups water
2/3 cup pickling salt
16 cloves garlic, peeled
8 heads fresh dill weed

Wash cucumbers and place in a tub of cold water and ice cubes. Soak for at least two hours, adding more ice as needed to keep them nice and cold. Make your brine by combining the vinegar, water, and pickling salt in a large saucepan. Bring to a full rolling boil.

Prepare sterilized quart jars. Place two cloves of garlic and one head of dill into each jar. Pack cucumbers into the jar. Carefully pour hot brine over cucumbers, leaving half an inch of headspace in the jar. Clean rims and seal jars with fresh, clean canning lids. Process sealed jars in a boiling water bath for fifteen minutes. Cool jars and put them away for about eight weeks before using.

Fermented Pickles and Sauerkraut

Fermented foods require salt for preservation and work well on both cabbage and cucumbers. For sauerkraut or fermented pickles, a 2–3 percent salt solution is used. Fermentation takes up to six weeks, during which the naturally occurring sugars in the vegetables are turned to lactic acid.

Sauerkraut can be made and canned in one step, or you can use the old-fashioned crock method.

Sauerkraut in a Crock

Clean and rinse cabbage and remove any damaged outer leaves. Cut the head into quarters and remove the core. Shred cabbage into long, thin shreds. For every five pounds of shredded cabbage, sprinkle in 3 tablespoons of pickling salt, mixing well to incorporate the salt throughout. Let the cabbage sit for ten minutes or until it begins to wilt.

Pack cabbage into a crock one layer at a time, tamping it down firmly after each layer until juices cover the top. Fill to within four inches of the top of the crock. There should be at least an inch of juice on top.

Take a large food-grade clear plastic bag and fill it with salted water. Place the bag on top of the cabbage so that it spreads out and covers the cabbage completely. Set the crock in an out-of-the-way place at room temperature. Check the kraut daily for signs of mold or scum. If it appears, just skim it off and discard. This is a normal part of the process. The sauerkraut will be ready in three to four weeks. It can now be canned or frozen for long-term storage.

Refrigerator Pickles

These pickles are generally brined in a mixture of salt and spices and refrigerated for several days before eating. While delicious, the acid level of these pickles is generally not quite high enough for long-term storage, but they do make a tasty side dish and will keep up to a couple of months. My refrigerator has a big jar of refrigerator pickles all summer long, and I keep it going by adding sliced cucumbers and brine as it gets depleted.

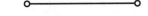

Refrigerator Pickles

2 pounds cucumbers, thinly sliced
2 cups onion, thinly sliced
1½ cups white vinegar
3/4 cup sugar
3/4 teaspoon salt
½ teaspoon mustard seed
½ teaspoon celery seed
½ teaspoon ground turmeric
¼ teaspoon black pepper
2 garlic cloves, thinly sliced

Alternate layers of cucumbers and onion in a large glass container. Place vinegar, sugar, and seasonings in a saucepan and bring to a boil, stirring to blend. Cook for one minute. Pour the hot liquid over the cucumber and onions. Refrigerate and let sit for four days before using.

Relish

A relish is any combination of chopped vegetables that have been cooked together in a vinegar solution. Pickle relish is the most common, but there are delicious corn, tomato, and other relish recipes. This onion relish is great on hamburgers or roasted pork.

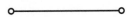

Onion Relish

3 tablespoons vegetable oil
12 cups white onions, chopped

1 cup celery, chopped
1 cup sugar
1 cup cider vinegar
½ cup water
½ teaspoon salt
1 teaspoon celery seed

Sauté onions and celery in oil until they are soft. Stir in sugar, vinegar, water, and spices and bring to a boil. Reduce heat and simmer gently for about twenty minutes, stirring occasionally. Let cool and refrigerate.

Fruit Pickles

Fruit pickles are made with tangy sweet-sour syrup. Pickled apples and spiced peaches make a wonderful accompaniment to roasted meat or chicken.

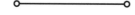

Pickled Peaches

8 pounds of peaches, peeled and halved
4 cups white vinegar
2 cups water
8 cinnamon sticks

Wash and peel peaches and cut them in half. As you work, place peeled peaches into a bowl of cold water and lemon juice to prevent them from darkening. Set aside until ready to use.

Make syrup by combining sugar, vinegar, water, and cinnamon sticks in a large saucepan. Bring mixture to a boil and then reduce heat and simmer for about thirty minutes.

Drain peaches and add them to the hot syrup. Return the syrup to a boil, and then reduce heat and continue to simmer for another twenty minutes. Remove cinnamon sticks. Pack hot peaches into pint canning jars and process for twenty minutes in a water bath canner.

Pickled Eggs

Make a brine of equal parts white vinegar and water along with one tablespoon of pickling salt for each cup of liquid, keeping it at a low boil while you prepare your jars. Place any seasonings that you may like in your brine. We usually add a bit of hot chili pepper, but dill, mustards, and even ginger make interesting choices.

Fill a quart jar with about twelve peeled hard-boiled eggs. Pour the hot brine over the eggs, wipe the rim, and seal with lid and ring. Process for twenty minutes in a water bath canner.

o———————o

Drying Fruits and Vegetables

Start with fresh, healthy ripened produce. Remove any produce that is past its prime or shows signs of bruising or other damage.

To sun-dry produce:

If your climate provides hot, sunny conditions and relatively low humidity for most of the day, consider sun-drying your produce.

Cut fruit into uniformly sized pieces. Fruit will darken as it dries, so pre-soak it in an ascorbic acid solution before you place it on drying racks. To make fruit leather, follow a recipe for a fruit purée and then pour purée onto plastic wrap-lined sheet trays and dry as you would fruit slices.

You can use a window screen as your drying rack if you like. Place fruit cut side down and lay out in the sun as early in the day as you can so you can take advantage of the most sun. A porch roof or a truck bed is ideal and will concentrate the heat to make drying much faster. A solar oven will also produce concentrated heat.

Cover racks with a light mesh fabric. Allow produce to dry on one side all day. At night, cover the screens with a light sheet, or bring everything inside if you think the evening will be cool or damp. The next day, turn produce over and repeat the process. Sun drying may take up to three days to complete. Dried fruit should be leathery but still flexible.

Most vegetables are best sliced as thin chips. When vegetables are clean and sliced, blanch them lightly in boiling water before beginning the drying process. This helps set the color and preserve many of the vitamins. When vegetables are ready, lay them out and dry as you would fruit.

To oven-dry produce:

In cooler or more humid conditions, oven-drying provides a more reliable method for producing consistently good dried fruit and vegetables.

Turn oven onto the lowest heat, about 200°F. Slice produce, stemming and removing seeds if necessary. Place on cookie sheets and leave in the oven all day or overnight. Check them occasionally, rotating sheets and turning over slices as needed. Larger pieces can take as much as forty-eight hours to reach the perfect dryness, but most will be done within twenty-four hours.

Dehydrators can also be used for drying. Dehydrators require electricity and relatively low capacity, but are very convenient for processing small batches.

Making Jerky

Start with two pounds of lean cut meat, like sirloin or a round steak. (It will be easier to work with if you freeze it slightly.) Trim all visible fat; lean jerky will keep better than fatty strips. Slice into very thin strips. Cut against the grain for a more tender jerky, with the grain for a chewier style.

If you want to flavor your meat, marinate it using a recipe created for jerky. I like soy sauce with garlic, salt, and just a dash of Tabasco, but this step is optional and I often skip it.

A good rub is important though. My rub consists of 2 teaspoons kosher salt, 1 teaspoon of black pepper, 1 teaspoon of garlic powder, and 1 tablespoon of brown sugar. Add some cayenne if you want a little kick. Coat your meat with this rub and refrigerate for twelve to twenty-four hours.

Another way to prepare your jerky is to combine your rub spices with your marinade. Marinate overnight and then dry your jerky. Check out jerky recipes and try one that sounds good to you.

Place your prepared meat on a broiler pan or a wire rack over a sheet tray, and place inside an oven set at about 200°F (a little lower if your oven setting goes below 200). Watch it carefully. If the heat is too low, it won't kill the bacteria. If it is too high, it will cook the meat rather than drying it out. If you have a dehydrator, follow the manufacturer's instructions.

Bake for four to six hours, or until jerky is dry to the touch and has a nice dark brown color inside. Cool at room temperature and store in sealable plastic bags.

Keeping Chickens

If you want to have a steady supply of eggs and are not squeamish about processing your own meat, you may find that raising chickens is a rewarding addition to your sustainable lifestyle.

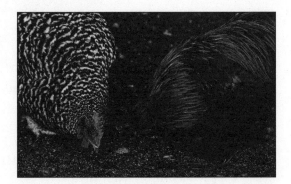

Backyard eggs contain one-third the cholesterol of store bought eggs, and more vitamin A, vitamin E, beta carotene, and Omega 3. Home-grown eggs are much more flavorful and richly colored than anything you will find in the grocery store. A family of four needs only a small flock to provide all the eggs it can use.

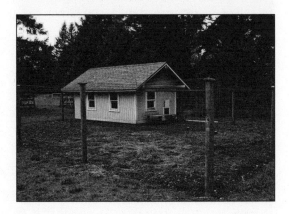

You can start your own chicken flock by buying chicks at the local feed store or farm supplier. The first sixty days are crucial. Young chicks need to be kept warm and be given clean bedding and a safe place to get some fresh air. After sixty days or when your chicks are feathered out, it is time to move them into a coop. Your chicken coop should be designed to protect chickens from weather and predators. There should be perches comfortable for roosting. You should plan on about two to three square feet of indoor space for each chicken and four to five square feet of outdoor run space per chicken.

Before embarking on a chicken project, get to know others in the area that raise chickens, and read up on all the ins-and-outs of being a chicken farmer. You may find that raising chickens may lead to you branching out and also raising goats and rabbits and your own honey bees.

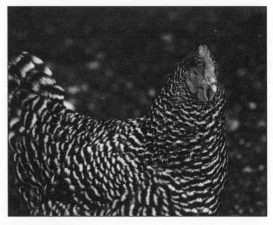

Or you may discover that raising chickens is not for you, but at least you'll meet others with whom you can barter for fresh eggs and organic meat.

Storing Fresh Farm Eggs without Refrigeration

Eggs are often used for bartering because chickens generally produce more than one family can use. But there is a way to store them in the pantry for use throughout the year.

Coat fresh, previously unrefrigerated eggs individually in a thick lard. Pack your eggs into a bucket, layering them with salt as you go. Place a tight lid on the bucket, label it with the date the eggs were laid, and store away in a cool, dark place. It is said that eggs stored this way will last up to one year, although I have never kept them that long.

There are three ways to tell whether eggs are still good for consumption. First, a good uncooked egg will never float to the surface in a bowl of cold water. It is okay if it bobbles or tips a bit. Second, if you shake an egg and listen, you should not hear anything. If you hear sloshing liquid, the egg is bad. Lastly, when you crack the egg, it will have a firm yolk and albumen that holds together. If it is very runny, the egg is bad.

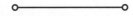

Keeping Honey Bees

If the idea of harvesting fresh honey straight from your own hive is appealing, consider establishing your own apiary. Raising bees is a relatively easy hobby with low start-up costs. Before considering raising bees, however, make sure regulations in your area allow you to establish hives and that your conditions are conducive to their needs. And be prepared for a few stings along the way! This is a natural part of bee keeping, so if anyone in your family is allergic to bee stings, you might want to skip this hobby.

The really beautiful thing about keeping bees is that, besides the honey and wax you get, bee pollinating habits can be very helpful to your fruit, vegetable, or nut crops. If you have a good location available in proximity to an orchard, berry bushes, a field of clover, or even a large garden, you may find keeping bees a nice complementary activity. Just make sure the environment is managed naturally; you do not want to expose your bees to excessive pesticides.

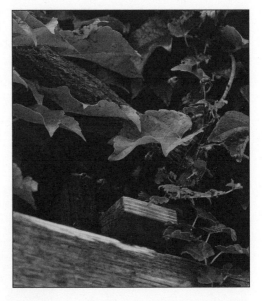

Honey bees want a location that is neither too warm nor too hot, and prefer a sheltered spot away from wind and excessive moisture. They will need a constant and reliable source of water, as well as a reliable supply of available nectar. You will need hives for the bees to live in, and can construct your own or buy pre-assembled models. In addition, you will want the appropriate protective gear, a smoker, and a couple of hand tools for harvesting honey and wax.

Once you introduce your bees to the hive, you may find that the first year requires a fair amount of watching and waiting. You will want to learn the habits of your bees so you know the times of greatest activity and pollen collection. Your honey harvest probably won't be very good the first year,

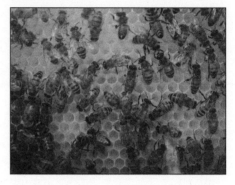

but once your hives are established, they should provide honey for years to come.

○──────────○

Growing Mushrooms

For those who have not taken the time to learn about them, mushrooms may seem like a bland, flavorless category of food. But they are actually power-packed little dynamos, with plenty of fiber and a number of essential vitamins and minerals. One Portobello mushroom equals the potassium from a whole banana and contains hard-to-get minerals such as iron, copper, zinc, and selenium. And because of their relatively mild flavor, you can use them as a replacement for meat in all kinds of dishes.

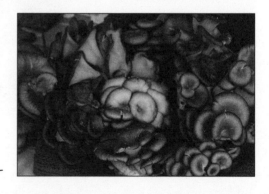

Growing mushrooms is one of the easiest projects you may ever do. All they really want is the proper hosting conditions and a little moisture.

There are a number of mushroom growing kits available on the market—a good option for learning the basics. But if you want to make your own, all you need are a log, a drill, and a couple of starting materials.

Shiitake mushrooms are fairly easy to grow. Buy mushroom plugs from a reputable supplier. These plugs are dowels that have been inoculated with mushroom spores. Choose a nice oak log that is four to six inches in diameter. Mushrooms get their nutrients from digesting wood, so you want a log that is dead, but not decomposing. Drill holes in the log along the top. Your hole should be just big enough for the mushroom plug to fit snugly and flush with the surface of the log. Paint over the holes with melted wax. Place your log in a shady location and water it every couple of weeks. Then wait! Fruiting takes place naturally after a heavy late spring or fall rain.

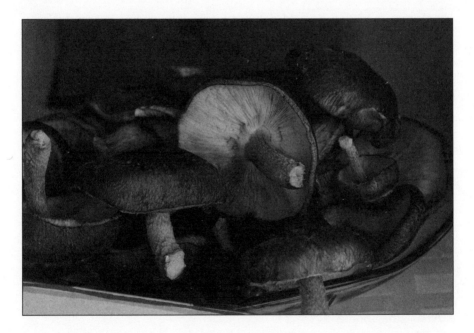

Mushrooms will grow in coffee grounds and some will grow on a bed of wood chips. With hundreds of different types of mushrooms available, there are a lot of options, so do your research before starting out. If you would like to be guided through your first experiment in mushroom growing, there are kits available that provide everything you need.

o———————o

Foraging

When all else fails, we can go back to getting food the way our ancestors did: by foraging the wild for them. While this may be somewhat impractical as a steady source of food, it can be an interesting and rewarding hobby, and will allow you to get to know your local flora on an intimate basis. CAUTION: It is very important that you educate yourself about your local foods. Learn the plants in your area and understand the safe places to gather them. Roadsides, for example, are exposed to road run-off and are often treated with pesticides. Buy a local guide to your area, and if possible, learn from an experienced forager. When in doubt, particularly with mushrooms, it is better to skip it until you are certain what you are picking.

Become accustomed to the rhythms of nature. Spring is the time for wild greens and mushrooms, late summer and early fall for fruits and nuts. Understand the food you are collecting. A tender fiddlehead becomes a bitter, indigestible green if picked too late. Acorns are a great source of nut meal, but only when carefully processed to leech out the bitter tannins. Start with the easy things, like dandelions, cattails, and nettles before going on to more adventurous choices.

Cattails are loaded with nutrition and are pretty easy to identify. The shoots can be harvested and used in a number of ways. After the outer leaves have been removed, the tender edible shoot is the texture of summer squash. They can be eaten raw in salads, stir-fried, or sautéed lightly and served with lemon and butter.

o———————o

Baked Cattail Casserole

2 cups peeled shoots, chopped
1 small onion, diced
1 cup bread crumbs
½ cup cheddar cheese, shredded

1 egg, beaten
½ cup milk
Salt and pepper to taste
2 tablespoons melted butter

Place cattail and onion in a saucepan with a little water. Cover and cook until slightly tender, about five minutes. Drain vegetables and combine in a bowl with bread crumbs and cheese. Whisk together egg and milk and add it to the bowl along with the melted butter. If you would like a golden brown topping, sprinkle the casserole with more bread crumbs and dot with a bit more butter. Bake at 350°F for about thirty minutes.

The following represent a few of the foods that can be found growing in the wild or on abandoned homesteads. If you have an interest in foraging, check your local extension office or find a book by a foraging expert to learn about the edibles in your area.

Edible Greens and Herbs

Bee balm
Chickweed
Chicory
Curly dock
Dandelion
Fiddlehead fern
Lamb's quarters
Nettle
Plantain
Pokeweed
Purslane
Sorrel
Watercress
Wild mustard

Edible Roots and Tubers

American lotus
Burdock
Cattail
Jerusalem artichoke
Ramps

Wild Mushrooms

Black trumpet
Chanterelle
Hen of the woods
Morel
Oyster

Wild Fruit

Blackberry
Blueberry
Chokeberry
Currants
Elderberry
Gooseberry
Mulberry
Pawpaw
Raspberry
Rose hips
Serviceberry
Wild cherry
Wild grapes
Wild plum
Wild strawberry

Nuts and Seeds

Acorn
Beechnut
Black walnut
Butternut
Hickory
Pecan
Pine nut
Sunflower
Wild rice

10

Home Remedies from the Family Pantry

Modern medicine is generally limited to the tests that doctors can recommend or the prescriptions they can provide. But the reality is that for most of the common little problems that come up day to day, our grandmothers probably know more about treating them than our doctor does.

Here are a few tried and true methods for dealing with tummy aches, head colds, and other kinds of aches and pains.

Caution: Sometimes the best course of treatment can only be provided by your physician. If symptoms are intense or last more than a few days, seek medical attention.

Keep Germs at Bay

Keeping yourself healthy is the first, and best, home remedy of all. Make sure you do not expose yourself unnecessarily to anything that could make you sick. The very best way to reduce or prevent the spread of illness is to keep your hands clean. Germs accumulate on your hands as you go through your day, and even the most innocent of objects may carry your next cold.

Hand Sanitizer

Instead of the store-bought version, it is easy to make your own hand sanitizer. Combine two cups of rubbing alcohol with one cup of aloe vera gel. I prefer mine to be unscented, but if you like, add a couple of drops of your favorite essential oil for a little fragrance.

How to Wash Your Hands

- Wet hands with warm water and add soap.
- Rub your hands together for about twenty seconds, making sure to scrub all surfaces, including back of hand, between fingers, wrists, and under nails. (This is about as long as it takes to sing Happy Birthday twice.)
- Rinse hands thoroughly with warm running water.
- If you are in a public location, dry your hands with a paper towel. Use that towel to turn off water and open the door before discarding.
- If water is not available, use a hand sanitizer that contains at least 60 percent alcohol. Your hands may not actually be clean, but at least you will have killed some germs.

Colds

There is an old saying that it takes two days to get a cold, three days to have a cold, and two days to get rid of a cold. There is no way to actually get rid of it, but there are a number of things you can do to make yourself more comfortable. Drink plenty of fluids to loosen phlegm and flush toxins out of your system. Use a humidifier to moisten the air in your home, and try a eucalyptus rub to ease congestion. And don't forget the chicken soup.

Certain foods can increase mucous production and should be avoided while you have a cold. Milk and dairy products are particular culprits, but wheat and even orange juice can have a negative effect on some people.

Clogged Sinuses

Clogged sinuses cause severe headaches and can lead to sinus infections if they go on too long. So get out the hot chili peppers! A hot, spicy meal will open up the sinuses and cause them to drain.

Sore Throat

Gargle with salt water to ease a sore throat, or try gargling with a 1:1 mix of water and lemon juice.

Asthma

For mild symptoms of asthma, drink a cup or two of strong coffee. It may not be a permanent substitute for medication, but it may provide some temporary relief.

Allergies

Use a simple saline solution to remove irritants in the nose. Make your own saline by mixing a teaspoon of salt and a pinch of baking soda in a pint of warm water.

Canker Sore

Place a dab of alum on a new canker sore to nip it in the bud. A mouthwash of goldenseal tea may also help it heal more quickly.

Indigestion

I always reached for an over-the-counter antacid whenever I found myself feeling bloated or a large meal left my stomach feeling acidic. Imagine my surprise when a friend suggested vinegar. Drink one tablespoon of vinegar when your stomach starts to fight you. It adds the acid that the stomach was working so hard to over-produce and settles your stomach very quickly. If the problem is a common one for you, add a tablespoon of vinegar to a glass of water and sip it with your meal.

For any kind of upset tummy, make a drink of chopped orange peel and water. Place the entire peel of one organic orange in a bowl. Pour two cups of boiling water over it and let steep until the water is completely cool.

Strain the tea and warm it up to your desired temperature. Sweeten it with honey, if you prefer.

Diarrhea

The most important thing to do when dealing with a bout of diarrhea is to stay hydrated. This is particularly important for little ones. A simple case of diarrhea can turn serious as they become dehydrated. Drink plenty of water and sip tea. Chamomile, red raspberry tea, and blackberry leaf tea are good herbal choices, but even the tannins in black tea can have a positive effect. Avoid dairy products as well as high fiber and greasy foods.

Constipation

To relieve constipation, mix two tablespoons of blackstrap molasses into a glass of warm milk or fruit juice. Drink before going to bed.

Diaper Rash

Use cornstarch instead of baby talc, which has added perfumes and other ingredients. Cornstarch can be applied to the bottom as well as to any of the creases and folds that may be susceptible to heat.

Burns

For minor burns, immediately get the affected area under cold running water. It doesn't have to be icy to reduce the pain. If you don't have running water, use a cold compress. If you have an aloe plant, break off a piece and apply its gel to the burn. Raw egg whites can also help relieve the pain.

Dry or Chapped Hands

Rub vegetable shortening into rough, dry hands and feet. Apply it in two thin layers. Rub in a small amount and then repeat with a second coating. Leave it on for a few minutes and then wipe off excess.

Sunburn

Pure aloe relieves the pain of a sunburn, but if a large portion of your body is affected, make a nice tea bath. Brew a strong tea by simmering several bags of black tea in a couple quarts of water for about 5 minutes. Pour the tea into a tepid bath and soak in it. An alternate approach is to make a sunburn spray by mixing equal parts olive oil and vinegar. Apply as needed to relieve pain.

Urinary Tract Infections

Cranberry juice and plenty of water will go a long way toward getting rid of a UTI. Flood your system with plenty of juice, or sip tea made from dried cranberries. I make a cranberry syrup when fresh cranberries are in season, specifically to use for wintertime tea.

Yeast Infections

A stomach bug or a large dose of antibiotics may sometimes clear the system of all those good bacteria that keep your gut in working order. Eat active-culture yogurt to help put those bacteria back in the system. For the little ones, just a tablespoon or two of yogurt a day will help them bounce back from a bout of the stomach flu.

Muscle Aches

Use ice packs immediately after an acute injury. Ice helps to reduce swelling and limit internal bleeding. Ice an injured joint for ten minutes at a time. Let the skin return to a normal temperature and then repeat the icing, up to three times. Do this for one to three days after an injury.

Use heat for chronic aching joints and stiffness. Heat is great for relaxing tight muscles and treating spasms. Use warm damp towels or warm therapy packs and leave them on the joint for fifteen to twenty minutes. Moist heat combined with eucalyptus ointment makes an especially comforting treatment. Just rub ointment on the joint, wrap in plastic wrap, and leave in place for about twenty minutes.

Bad Breath

To make an antiseptic mouthwash, mix one part hydrogen peroxide and one part water and rinse the mouth out. For a more pleasant tasting mouthwash, mix one cup of water with twenty to twenty-five drops of your favorite mint oil.

Athlete's Foot

Make a paste of baking soda and water. Rub into feet and between toes. Rinse and dry thoroughly.

Smelly Feet

Soak feet in a strong blend of salt and water; about four cups in one gallon of water. For best results, don't rinse or towel dry your feet after the soak. Just let them air dry.

Stings and Insect Bites

Bug bites and stings are no fun—pain, itching, and swelling are common, and some people have stronger reactions than others. If there is swelling, place ice on the sting immediately. When the swelling is under control, apply a paste of baking soda and water to reduce pain and itching. If the pain or itch is bad, try placing an aspirin directly on the bite, or applying a paste of aspirin and water.

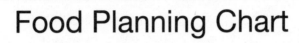

Food Planning Chart

ITEM	NUMBER ON HAND	SIZE	AMOUNT NEEDED FOR 3 MONTH SUPPLY	AMOUNT TO BUY
Sample - *canned black beans*	*6*	*15 OZ*	*24*	*18*
Water				
Grains				
Barley				
Dry corn				
Flax				
Flaxseed flour				
Millet				
Quinoa				
Rolled Oats				
Spelt flour				
Wheat				

ITEM	NUMBER ON HAND	SIZE	AMOUNT NEEDED FOR 3 MONTH SUPPLY	AMOUNT TO BUY
White flour				
Whole Wheat flour				
Rice				
Brown rice				
Converted rice				
White rice				
Wild rice				
Cereals				
Cream of wheat				
Dry cereal				
Granola				
Multi-grain cereal				
Oatmeal				
Pasta				
Couscous				
Egg noodles				
Elbow macaroni				
Orzo				
Spaghetti				
Legumes				
Black Beans				
Cannellini beans				

ITEM	NUMBER ON HAND	SIZE	AMOUNT NEEDED FOR 3 MONTH SUPPLY	AMOUNT TO BUY
Kidney Beans				
Lentils				
Lima Beans				
Navy beans				
Peanut butter powder				
Peanut butter, emulsified				
Peanut butter, natural				
Peanuts				
Pinto beans				
Split peas				
TVP				
Yellow peas				
Proteins				
Beef dices				
Chicken dices				
Ham dices				
Ham, canned				
Jerky				
Salmon, canned				
Sardines				
Sausage				

ITEM	NUMBER ON HAND	SIZE	AMOUNT NEEDED FOR 3 MONTH SUPPLY	AMOUNT TO BUY
Shrimp, canned				
Spam				
Tuna, canned				
Dairy and Eggs				
Butter powder				
Cheese, dried				
Dried eggs				
Dry milk				
Egg whites				
Sour cream powder				
Canned Vegetables				
Artichokes				
Asparagus				
Baked beans				
Beets				
Black beans				
Carrots				
Chiles, green				
Corn				
Green beans				
Kidney beans				
Mushrooms				
Olives				
Peas				

ITEM	NUMBER ON HAND	SIZE	AMOUNT NEEDED FOR 3 MONTH SUPPLY	AMOUNT TO BUY
Pinto beans				
Pumpkin				
Squash				
Tomato paste				
Tomato sauce				
Tomatoes, diced				
Yams				
Dried Vegetables				
Bell peppers				
Broccoli				
Cabbage				
Carrots				
Celery				
Chile peppers				
Corn				
Green beans				
Mushrooms				
Onions				
Peas				
Potato flakes				
Tomato powder				
Sprouting Seeds				
Alfalfa				
Chia				
Lentil				

ITEM	NUMBER ON HAND	SIZE	AMOUNT NEEDED FOR 3 MONTH SUPPLY	AMOUNT TO BUY
Mung				
Radish				
Soybeans				
Sunflower				
Canned Fruits				
Applesauce				
Apricots				
Blueberries				
Cherries				
Fruit cocktail				
Grapefruit				
Mandarin oranges				
Peaches				
Pears				
Pineapple				
Dried Fruits				
Apples				
Apricots				
Bananas				
Cranberries				
Dates				
Figs				
Mango				

ITEM	NUMBER ON HAND	SIZE	AMOUNT NEEDED FOR 3 MONTH SUPPLY	AMOUNT TO BUY
Prunes				
Raisins				
Baking Needs				
Baking powder				
Baking soda				
Cornmeal				
Cornstarch				
Cream of tartar				
Wheat for grinding				
White flour				
Yeast				
Sweeteners				
Brown sugar				
Corn syrup				
Honey				
Maple syrup				
Molasses				
Powdered sugar				
White sugar				
Fats				
Butter powder				
Cooking oil				
Shortening				
Shortening powder				

ITEM	NUMBER ON HAND	SIZE	AMOUNT NEEDED FOR 3 MONTH SUPPLY	AMOUNT TO BUY
Spices and Flavorings				
Basil				
Cayenne powder				
Chili powder				
Cinnamon				
Cloves				
Cocoa powder				
Dill				
Dry mustard				
Garlic powder				
Ginger				
Nutmeg				
Onion flakes				
Oregano				
Paprika				
Pepper				
Peppercorns				
Pickling spices				
Sage				
Salt				
Sesame seeds				
Thyme				
Vanilla				

ITEM	NUMBER ON HAND	SIZE	AMOUNT NEEDED FOR 3 MONTH SUPPLY	AMOUNT TO BUY
Sauces and Spice Blends				
Beef bouillon cubes				
Cheese sauce powder				
Chicken bouillon cubes				
Gravy mix				
Drink Mixes				
Apple cider powder				
Chocolate milk powder				
Coffee				
Lemonade				
Orange drink				
Tea				
Convenience Foods				
Baking mix				
Canned brown bread				
Cold cereal				
Instant rice				
Pancake mix				

ITEM	NUMBER ON HAND	SIZE	AMOUNT NEEDED FOR 3 MONTH SUPPLY	AMOUNT TO BUY
Snacks and Desserts				
Cake mix				
Gelatin				
Jams				
Pie filling				
Popcorn				
Pudding mix				
Canned Soups				
Beef stock				
Chicken noodle				
Chicken stock				
Cream of mushroom				
Potato				
Vegtable beef				
Condiments				
Barbecue sauce				
Ketchup				
Mayonnaise				
Mustard				
Pickles				
Salad dressing				
Salsa				
Soy sauce				

ITEM	NUMBER ON HAND	SIZE	AMOUNT NEEDED FOR 3 MONTH SUPPLY	AMOUNT TO BUY
Baby food				
Baby cereal				
Canned baby food				
Evaporated milk				
Formula				
Paper Products				
Aluminum foil				
Garbage bags				
Napkins				
Paper cups				
Paper plates				
Paper towels				
Plastic bags				
Plastic wrap				
Toilet paper				
Cleansers				
Ammonia				
Bathroom cleaner				
Bleach				
Dish soap				
Floor cleaner				
Glass cleaner				

ITEM	NUMBER ON HAND	SIZE	AMOUNT NEEDED FOR 3 MONTH SUPPLY	AMOUNT TO BUY
Laundry soap				
Multi-purpose cleaner				
Scrub brushes				
Personal Hygiene				
Bar soap				
Body lotion				
Cotton swabs				
Deodorant				
Feminine hygiene products				
Hair conditioner				
Razors				
Shampoo				
Shaving cream				
Toothpaste				
First Aid				
Adhesive bandages				
Aloe cream for sunburns				
Antacids				
Antibiotics				

ITEM	NUMBER ON HAND	SIZE	AMOUNT NEEDED FOR 3 MONTH SUPPLY	AMOUNT TO BUY
Anti-diarrheal medicine				
Antihistamines				
Aspirin				
Burn ointment				
Cold medicine				
Elastic bandages				
Epsom Salt				
First aid tape				
Gauze				
Hot and cold packs				
Hydrogen Peroxide				
Ibuprophen				
Laxatives				
Multi-Vitamins				
Painkiller				
Petroleum jelly				
Prescription medicines				
Rubbing Alcohol				
Small scissors				

ITEM	NUMBER ON HAND	SIZE	AMOUNT NEEDED FOR 3 MONTH SUPPLY	AMOUNT TO BUY
Small splints				
Sterile cotton balls				
Sunscreen				
Syrup of ipecac				
Thermometer				
Triple antibiotic cream				
Tweezers				
Tylenol				

Family Pantry and Emergency Resources

Shelf Reliance
691 South Auto Mall Drive
American Fork, UT 84003
801-756-9902
www.shelfreliance.com

The Wise Food Supply Company
8899 S 700 E
Sandy, UT 84070
888-406-2080
www.wisefoodsupply.com

Solar Oven Society
1754 Terrace Drive
Roseville, MN 55113
612-623-4700
www.solarovens.org

Lodge Manufacturing
South Pittsburg, TN
423-837-7181
www.lodgemfg.com

Emergency Essentials
653 North 1500 West
Orem, UT 84057
800-999-1863
www.beprepared.com

SOS Survival Products
15705 Strathern Street, #11
Van Vuys, CA 91406
800-479-7998
www.sosproduct.com

Grainger
100 Grainger Parkway
Lake Forest, IL 60045
800-323-0620
www.grainger.com

Brunton Outdoor
2255 Brunton Court
Riverton, WY 82501 USA
307-857-4700
www.bruntonoutdoor.com

eGear
Revere Supply Company
7720 Philips Highway
Jacksonville, FL 32256
877-738-3738
www.egear.com

Yellowstone Trading Company
PO Box 3235
Bozeman, MT 59772
406-586-8248
www.yellowstonetrading.com

SproutPeople
170 Mendell St.
San Francisco, CA 94124
877-777-6887
www.sproutpeople.com